This publication is designed to provide accurate and authoritative information in regard to the subject matter covered. It is sold with the understanding that neither the author nor the publisher is engaged in rendering legal, investment, accounting or other professional services. While the publisher and author have used their best efforts in preparing this book, they make no representations or warranties with respect to the accuracy or completeness of the contents of this book and specifically disclaim any implied warranties of merchantability or fitness for a particular purpose. No warranty may be created or extended by sales representatives or written sales materials. The advice and strategies contained herein may not be suitable for your situation. You should consult with a professional when appropriate. Neither the publisher nor the author shall be liable for any loss of profit or any other commercial damages, including but not limited to special, incidental, consequential, personal, or other damages.

THE IMMUNE SYSTEM BOOK: HOW TO MAXIMIZE YOUR BODY'S NATURAL DEFENSES

By

Alexander Wright

Table of Contents

CHAPTER 1: EXERCISE

While there are multiple ways to boost immunity, exercise is one of the most effective and natural ways to do so. Exercise not only helps improve physical health but also plays a crucial role in enhancing your immune system. We will dive into the science behind how exercise helps boost immunity, different types of exercises that optimize your immune system, and tips on how to incorporate exercise into your daily routine. We will also discuss the frequency of exercise required for optimal immune health and whether too much exercise can weaken the immune system. So, let's get moving towards a healthier immune system!

The Connection Between Exercise and Immunity

Regular physical activity can enhance immune health by improving the body's immune response and strengthening immune system cells and function. Exercise also reduces the risk of infection by boosting immune function and lowering stress hormones. Studies have shown that aerobic exercise, such as brisk walking or cycling, can lead to a brief rise in body temperature, which can prevent bacterial growth, and form a first line of defense against infections. Maintaining healthy levels of physical activity is a great way to support your mental health, while reducing the risk of infection during flu season.

The Science Behind Exercise and Immunity

Stimulating the immune system, exercise

enhances overall health and increases its functions. It optimizes cellular immunity and helps flush bacteria, reducing infection risk. Adequate exercise can lower viral infection risk, emphasizing its crucial role in immune health. Studies show that physical activity plays a significant role in improving immune response, especially during flu season. The release of stress hormones is reduced through exercise, benefiting mental health and the immune system. Exercise supports healthy immune function by improving blood flow, lymphatic system circulation, and white blood cell activity.

Optimizing Immune System Through Different Types of Exercises

Walking promotes overall health by enhancing immunity, while strength training contributes to improved immune health. Additionally, high-intensity interval training strengthens the immune system and varying exercise routines can support overall immune function. Different types of exercises play a crucial role in boosting the immune system, from promoting the release of stress hormones to improving mental health. Moreover, studies suggest that different forms of exercise can lead to a lower risk of infection and help in optimizing the innate immune system. The combination of various types of exercises is a great way to maintain a healthy immune system during flu season.

Walking for Immunity Enhancement

Taking brisk walks enhances the circulation of immune cells, supporting overall immune health and reducing the risk of infection. Regular walks aid in the functions of the immune system, contributing to overall immune function improvement. Studies have shown that walking lowers the risk of common cold infections, making it a great way to support a healthy immune system during flu season. Additionally, walking can also contribute to mental health and release of stress hormones, further enhancing the body's ability to fight off infections.

Strength Training and Immune Health

Engaging in strength training promotes immune system health, supporting overall wellness. Regular strength training sessions benefit immune function by lowering the risk of infection. Studies indicate that resistance workouts contribute to immune system strength and enhance overall immune health. The systematic review published in the British Journal of Sports Medicine supports the positive impact of strength training on a healthy immune system. Additionally, promoting the release of stress hormones through strength training can also positively impact mental health and the body's innate immune system.

High-Intensity Interval Training (HIIT) for a Stronger Immune System

Stimulating immune function, HIIT benefits overall health by promoting immune system health and enhancing its functions. Studies show that HIIT helps lower the risk of infection, making it effective in supporting overall immune health. The release of stress hormones during intense exercise positively impacts mental health, while the brief rise in body temperature supports the healthy functioning of the immune system. Incorporating HIIT into your routine can be a great way to support your immune system, especially during flu season. Studies of people engaging in vigorous intensity exercises like HIIT have shown a lower risk of infection, as published in the British Journal of Sports Medicine.

Frequency of Exercise for Immune Health Improvement

Balancing the frequency of exercise is crucial for maintaining a healthy immune system. Consistent, moderate physical activity has been shown to boost immune function, supporting overall wellness. The duration of exercise also plays a role in impacting the strength of the immune system. Studies emphasize the importance of exercising consistently to improve immune health. Finding the right balance in the frequency and duration of exercise sessions is key to supporting the body's immune functions and overall well-being.

Consistency and Duration of Exercise Sessions

Balancing the frequency and duration of exercise is key to enhancing immune health. Regardless of duration, consistent exercise contributes to overall immune system strength. Longer, regular exercise sessions specifically support immune system functions, aiding in the release of stress hormones and promoting mental health. Studies emphasize the impactful role of exercise consistency on immunity, highlighting its potential to lower the risk of infection during flu season. Finding the right balance between exercise duration and frequency is essential for maintaining a healthy immune system and optimizing overall well-being.

Balancing Exercise Frequency to Avoid Immunity Suppression

Over-exercising can lead to weakened immune function, so balancing exercise frequency helps avoid immune system suppression. Studies caution against excessive exercise's impact on immunity and highlight the importance of maintaining a balanced exercise routine to support immune health. Finding a healthy balance in exercise frequency not only benefits immune health but also contributes to overall well-being. It's essential to consider the type of exercise and its intensity, as this can impact the immune system. Consistency in exercise frequency and duration plays a crucial role in supporting immune system functions.

Can Too Much Exercise Weaken the Immune System?

Excessive exercise can weaken the immune system. High-intensity workouts may temporarily lower immunity, increasing the risk of infection. Striking a balance between exercise and rest is crucial for maintaining a strong immune system. Moderate exercise supports immune function without compromising it.

Tips for Incorporating Exercise into Your Routine

Regular physical activity is essential for overall health, including a strong immune system. Aim to engage in at least 150 minutes of moderate exercise each week, incorporating both strength training and aerobic activities. It's important to stay active throughout the day to support immune function. Finding physical activities that you enjoy will make exercise a regular and enjoyable habit. By doing so, you contribute to the promotion of your overall health, including immune function, and improve mental well-being.

Conclusion

Regular exercise plays a crucial role in boosting your immune system. It helps strengthen the body's defense mechanisms, reduces the risk of chronic diseases, and improves overall health and well-being. Whether it's walking, strength training, or high-intensity interval training (HIIT), incorporating different types of exercises into your routine can optimize your immune system. However, it's important to find the right balance. Consistency and duration of exercise sessions are key, but too much exercise can weaken your immune system. It's important to listen to your body and avoid overexertion. By making exercise a regular part of your routine and following these tips, you can support your immune system and enjoy the benefits of improved health and vitality.

CHAPTER 2: DIET

A healthy diet plays a vital role in keeping your immune system functioning well. We will explore the link between diet and immunity. We will cover the nutrients that are essential for boosting your immune system, as well as the detrimental effects of a poor diet on your immunity. Additionally, we will dive into diets that can help boost your immunity, their benefits, and limitations. Lastly, we have listed down some essential foods that you can incorporate into your diet to enhance your immunity. Read on to discover which foods can help give your immune system a much-needed boost!

Understanding the Connection Between Diet and Immune System

A well-balanced diet profoundly influences the health of the immune system. Critical vitamins and essential nutrients are vital for maintaining a strong immunity. Consistent nourishment plays a pivotal role in supporting the body's defense mechanisms. Additionally, inadequate sleep can detrimentally impact the body's immune response. Overall well-being is intricately connected to a robust immune system. Deep sleep also contributes significantly to the body's immune function by allowing it to rest and repair.

The Role of Nutrients in Immune Health

Adequate intake of essential vitamins, such as vitamin C and vitamin D, is crucial for supporting immunity.

Additionally, zinc plays a vital role in the proper functioning of the immune system. Moreover, antioxidants are key players in maintaining optimal immune health. It's important to note that nutrition directly influences the body's immune response, while specific nutrients actively support white blood cells in their fight against pathogens. Deep sleep also contributes to immune function, further emphasizing the interconnectedness of various factors in bolstering the body's defense mechanisms.

Detrimental Effects of a Poor Diet on Immunity

The repercussions of a poor diet on the immune system can lead to adverse effects. Inflammation, which is a common outcome of a poor diet, can significantly impact immune health and weaken the body's defense mechanisms. Furthermore, diets lacking in essential nutrients can compromise the immune system's ability to ward off illnesses, making the body more susceptible to infections. Additionally, smoking not only compromises immune health but also increases the vulnerability to flu and other respiratory infections. Moreover, the absence of relaxation techniques can have a detrimental impact on overall health, including immunity. Prioritizing relaxation and incorporating beneficial foods like sauerkraut and legumes into one's diet is crucial for maintaining and enhancing immune health.

Diets That Boost the Immune System

Strengthening the immune response is achievable through immune-boosting diets. It is essential to incorporate flu-fighting foods into the diet to bolster immunity. The most effective way to enhance immunity is by consuming a nutritious diet, while also considering the role of meditation and yoga in aiding immune health. Additionally, including immune-boosting ingredients in the diet is crucial for optimal immune function. Deep sleep is vital for immune health and overall well-being, making it a key aspect to consider when focusing on diets that boost the immune system.

Overview of Immune-Boosting Diets

Supporting immune health through dietary choices is crucial. The Mediterranean diet, renowned for its health benefits, has been linked to improved immune function. Additionally, plant-based diets are rich in essential nutrients that promote a robust immune system. Incorporating probiotics and prebiotics into the diet can also play a vital role in strengthening immunity. Furthermore, emphasizing regular nourishment through immune-boosting diets is key to maintaining optimal immune function. Adopting a balanced diet, abundant in nutrients and vitamins, is essential for overall immune health and well-being.

Benefits and Limitations of These Diets

Immune-boosting diets play a crucial role in providing essential nutrition for the immune system, contributing to good health and immunity. However, it's important to note that some of these diets may have limitations and require careful consideration. Consistency in following these diets is key to their effectiveness in combating germs and strengthening the immune system. Additionally, the emphasis on regular nourishment through these diets is vital for maintaining a healthy immune response. While the benefits are evident, it's essential to be mindful of any potential limitations and ensure a balanced approach to reaping the full advantages of immune-boosting diets.

Essential Foods to Enhance Immunity

Strengthening the body's defense system through nutrition is crucial for overall well-being. Including vital components, such as immune-boosting supplements, in your daily intake can be highly beneficial. It's essential to consume foods rich in immune-boosting properties to support good health, as the diet plays a significant role in enhancing immunity. By incorporating key nutrients and essential vitamins into your meals, you can effectively enhance your body's ability to combat germs and stay healthy. Deep sleep also contributes to improved immune function, making it an essential aspect of maintaining a robust immune system.

What Makes These Foods Effective for Immune Support?

The effectiveness of immune-boosting foods lies in their ability to aid antibody production and strengthen the immune system. These essential foods contain key nutrients that support a healthy immune response, ultimately enhancing overall immune health.

Conclusion

In conclusion, maintaining a healthy immune system is crucial for overall well-being and disease prevention. A nutrient-rich diet plays a significant role in boosting immunity and protecting against illnesses. Incorporating immune-boosting foods into your daily meals can provide essential vitamins, minerals, and antioxidants that enhance the functioning of your immune system. Foods such as citrus fruits, leafy greens, garlic, ginger, and yogurt are known for their immune-boosting properties. However, it's important to note that relying solely on specific foods may not be sufficient. A balanced diet, regular exercise, adequate sleep, and stress management are equally important for a strong immune system. Prioritize your health by making conscious choices and taking care of your body.

CHAPTER 3: SLEEP

As mentioned in the previous chapter, the quality, duration, and consistency of your sleep affects every aspect of your health, including your immune system.

How Much Sleep Do We Need?

The amount of sleep differs based, first, on age. The general recommendations according to The National Center for Biotechnology Information are:

Age Group	Age Range	Recommended
Infant	4-12 months	12-16 hours
Toddler	1-2 years	11-14 hours
Preschool	3-5 years	0-13 hours
School-age	6-12 years	9-12 hours
Teen	13-18 years	8-10 hours
Adult	18 years and older	7-9 hours

This table does not include recommendations for newborns because their needs vary wildly, ranging anywhere from 11 hours to 19 hours per 24-hour period.

The American Academy of Sleep Medicine put together a group of experts on sleep to come up with these suggestions. The group members looked at hundreds of high-quality studies about the link between how long you sleep and important health issues like heart disease, depression, pain, and diabetes.

After looking at the facts, the group went through several rounds of voting and talking to narrow down the numbers for how much sleep different ages need. Other medical groups, like the Sleep Research Society, the American Academy of Pediatrics, and more, have agreed with the final suggestions.

It is essential to understand that these are general recommendations. You are an individual. As an individual, your needs may be different than others. Here are some things to consider that may have an impact on your individual needs. To figure out how much sleep you need, you must think about your overall health, the things you do every day, and how you usually sleep. Some things that can help you figure out how much sleep you need are:

Do you feel healthy, happy, and active after seven hours of sleep? Or, have you found that you need more sleep to really get going?

Do you have more than one health problem that might need you to rest more?

Do you use a lot of energy every single day? Do you play sports or have a job that requires a lot of physical work?

Do the things you do every day require you to be alert to do them safely? Do you drive a lot every day or use big equipment? Do any of these things ever make you feel sleepy?

Do you have trouble sleeping or have you had trouble sleeping in the past?

Does caffeine help you get through the day?

Do you tend to sleep in more when you have a lot of free time?

You can figure out how much sleep you need based on how you answer these questions.

Sleeping Too Much

While individual concerns are relevant, there is a limit. Most people know that getting too little sleep can hurt your health. Getting too little sleep on a regular basis is linked to several long-term diseases, as well as making you cranky and tired during the day. But did you know that sleeping too much can also be bad? Oversleeping is linked to several health issues, as well such as:

- Type 2 diabetes
- Heart trouble
- Obesity
- Depression
- Headaches

Does sleeping too much make you sick, or is it a sign of a problem you already have? Either way, you might want to see your doctor if you are always falling asleep or looking for the next nap.

If you need more than 8 or 9 hours of sleep every night to feel relaxed, this could be a sign of a deeper problem. Many things affect the quality of your sleep, making you feel tired and sluggish even after 8 hours in bed. Among these problems are:

- Sleep apnea
- Restless legs syndrome
- Bruxism (teeth grinding)
- Chronic pain
- Some prescription drugs

Then there are situations that don't change the quality of your sleep much but make you need more sleep. Among them are:

- Narcolepsy

- Delayed sleep phase syndrome
- Idiopathic hypersomnia

These problems can be treated, which can help you sleep better.

Many people think it's a normal part of aging that they need more sleep, but getting older shouldn't make a big difference in how much sleep you need.

If you've checked out those problems and you're still hitting the snooze button after 9 hours under the covers, it could be a sign that you have a heart problem, diabetes, or depression, and you should speak to a doctor. He or she might also suggest a sleep study to make sure there aren't any sleep problems.

Sleeping Too Little

Simply not getting enough sleep is referred to as sleep deprivation, but there is a broader concept known as "sleep deficiency," which encompasses sleep deprivation as well as other issues. Sleep deficiency can be caused by any of the following:

- You don't get enough sleep.
- You sleep at the wrong time of day.
- You don't sleep well or get all the different kinds of sleep your body needs.
- You have a sleep disorder that makes it hard for you to get enough sleep or makes the sleep you do get less restful.

People need to sleep just as much as they need to eat, drink, and breathe and is just as important to your health and happiness as these other things. About one-third of people in the United States don't get enough rest or sleep every day, according to the Centers for Disease Control and Prevention. Nearly 40% of people say they fall asleep during the day at least once a month when they didn't mean to. Also, between 50 and 70 million Americans have sleep problems that don't go away.

Lack of sleep can cause problems with your physical and mental health, accidents, less work output, and even a higher chance of dying. Lack of sleep can make it hard to do well at your job, school, driving, and with other people. You might find it hard to learn, pay attention, and move. Also, it might be hard for you to understand how other people feel and act. Lack of sleep can also make you feel angry, irritable, or worried around other people.

Children and adults may have different signs of not getting enough sleep. When kids don't get enough sleep, they might be overly active and have trouble paying attention. They might also misbehave, which can hurt how well they do in school.

Adults, teens, and kids who don't get enough sleep are also more likely to get hurt. For example, sleepiness while driving is a major cause of serious injuries and deaths in car accidents. When it comes to older people, not getting enough sleep may make them more likely to fall and break a bone. People who don't get enough sleep have also made mistakes that led to terrible accidents like nuclear plant meltdowns, big ships running aground, and plane crashes.

People often believe that they can get by with less sleep and nothing bad will happen. But studies show that getting enough good sleep at the right times is important for mental health, physical health, quality of life, and safety.

Science of Sleep

There are many things that help your body get ready to sleep and wake up. Your body has several internal clocks called circadian clocks. These typically follow a 24-hour repeating rhythm called the circadian rhythm. This rhythm affects every cell, tissue, and organ in your body.

Your central circadian clock, located in your brain, tells you when it is time for sleep. Other circadian clocks are in organs throughout your body. Your body's internal clocks are in sync with certain cues in the environment. Light, darkness, and other cues help determine when you feel awake and when you feel drowsy. Artificial light and caffeine can disrupt this process by giving your body false wakefulness cues.

Your body clock may not be the same as other people's. The natural circadian cycle of most people is a little longer than 24 hours. Some people wake up early by nature, while others stay up late by nature. For example, it's normal for many teenagers to want to go to bed later and wake up later.

With age, the rhythm and timing of body clocks also change. Neurons, or cells, that help you sleep are lost as a normal part of getting older. Some diseases, like Alzheimer's, can also speed up the death of neurons. This makes it harder for older people to sleep through the night. Circadian rhythms can also be changed by things like less physical activity or less time spent outside. Because of this, most older people sleep less and wake up earlier.

When you have been awake for a long time, your body's biological need for sleep grows. This is controlled by homeostasis, the process by which your body keeps your systems, like your internal body temperature, stable. This need to sleep is linked to a chemical called adenosine. The amount of adenosine in your brain keeps going up as long as you are awake. The shift toward sleep is shown by the rising levels. This process can be stopped by caffeine and other drugs that block adenosine.

If you follow the natural pattern of days and nights, your eyes send signals to your brain that it is daytime. The part of your brain that gets these signals is called the suprachiasmatic nucleus. The sympathetic system and the parasympathetic system send these signals to the rest of your body. This helps your body's main clock keep track of day and night. This process is messed up when people are exposed to artificial light.

The cycle of light and dark affects when your brain makes and releases melatonin. Your bloodstream carries melatonin to the cells in your body. Melatonin starts to build up in your bloodstream in the evening and reaches its highest level in the early morning. Melatonin is thought to help you fall asleep. When you're exposed to more light, like when the sun comes up, your body makes a chemical called cortisol. Cortisol helps your body get ready to wake up on its own.

If you are exposed to bright artificial light late at night, it can mess up this process and stop your brain from making melatonin. This can make it more difficult to go to sleep. Bright artificial light comes from things like a TV screen, a smartphone, or an alarm clock with a very bright light. Some people use physical filters or software to block some of the blue light from these devices.

Your central circadian clock is not always in sync with the time you go to sleep. Jet lag or night shifts can cause it to go out of sync.

When you sleep, you go back and forth between two stages: rapid eye movement (REM) sleep and non-REM sleep. Every 80 to 100 minutes, the cycle starts again. Most nights, there are four to six cycles. Between cycles, you might wake up for a short time.

Non-REM sleep has three stages:

Stage 1: This is the transition between being awake and going to sleep.

Stage 2: At this point, you are asleep.

Stage 3. This stage of sleep is called deep sleep or slow-wave sleep. You usually spend more time in this stage earlier in the night.

REM sleep is when your eyes twitch and your brain is active. Brain activity during REM sleep is about the same as brain activity when you are awake. REM sleep is when most people dream. Most of the time, your muscles weaken, preventing you from acting out your dreams. You typically have more REM sleep later in the night, but you don't get as much REM sleep in colder temperatures. This is because your body doesn't regulate your temperature properly during REM sleep.

As people get older, their sleep habits and types change. For example, babies spend more time in REM sleep. The amount of slow-wave sleep is highest when a child is young and drops sharply when he or she is a teenager. Slow-wave sleep gets less and less as people get older, and some older people may not have any at all.

The way you feel while you are awake depends in part on what happens while you are sleeping. During sleep, your body is working to support healthy brain function and maintain your physical health.

Children and teens also grow and develop better when they get enough sleep. It can also affect how well you think, act, work, learn, and get along with others.

When you fall asleep and go into non-REM sleep, your heart rate and blood pressure drop. During sleep, your body is controlled by your parasympathetic system, and your heart doesn't have to work as hard as it does when you're awake. Your sympathetic nervous system is turned on during REM sleep and when you wake up. This raises your heart rate and blood pressure to your usual levels when awake and calm.

People who don't get enough sleep or wake up often at night may be more likely to have:

- Coronary artery disease
- High blood pressure
- Obesity
- Stroke

At different times of the day, your body makes different

hormones. This may be related to your sleep patterns or circadian clocks. Your body makes hormones, like cortisol, that make you more awake in the morning. Other hormones have 24-hour cycles that change as you age. For example, in children, the hormones that tell the glands to release testosterone, estrogen, and progesterone are made in pulses at night, and the pulses get bigger as puberty approaches.

Different circadian clocks, such as those in the liver, fat, and muscle, affect how your body deals with fat. For example, these circadian clocks make sure that your liver is ready to help digest fat at the right times. If you eat at odd times, your body may handle fat in a different way.

Studies have shown that not getting enough good sleep can lead to:

- Higher levels of hunger-controlling hormones like leptin and ghrelin in your body.
- Less ability to respond to insulin.
- More eating, especially fatty, sweet, and salty foods.
- Decreased physical activity
- Metabolic Syndrome

And all these things can contribute to being overweight or obese.

During sleep, you take in less oxygen and breathe less often and less deeply. People with health problems like asthma or chronic obstructive pulmonary disease (COPD) may have trouble with these changes. Most of the time, asthma symptoms are worse in the early morning. People with lung diseases like COPD can also have trouble breathing that gets worse at night.

Sleep also affects your immune system. Different parts of your immune system are more active at different times of the day. For example, a certain type of immune cell works harder when you sleep. Because of this, people who don't get enough sleep may get colds and other infections more often.

Sleep helps with learning and the formation of long-term memories. If you don't get enough sleep or high-quality sleep, it can be more difficult to concentrate on tasks and think clearly.

Sleep Hygiene

Sleep hygiene may be the most talked about subject when it comes to sleep. Your sleep hygiene can make a pivotal difference to your sleep. Here are some of the most common and most effective do's and don't of sleep hygiene.

What to do:

- Try to sleep around the same time each night and wake up around the same time each morning.
- Exercise for at least 30 minutes a day, about five days a week. Exercise hard only in the morning or afternoon. Before bed, you can do more relaxing exercises, like yoga.
- Get a lot of sunlight. Open your blinds as soon as you wake up and spend some time outside at some point. You can also use a light box first thing in the morning on dark winter days to help your brain wake up and keep your body's rhythms in sync.
- Set up a regular, relaxing routine for going to bed.
- Take a warm shower or bath before you go to sleep.
- Do relaxation exercises like mindful breathing and progressive muscle relaxation before you go to sleep.
- Make sure the place where you sleep is nice and calm. Your room shouldn't be too hot, too cold, or too bright, and your bed should

be comfortable. Use earplugs and an eye mask if you feel the need. Make sure your pillow feels good.

- Reserve your bed for sleep and sex. Don't eat, watch TV, or work in bed.
- Go to bed when you're tired and get out of bed if you can't sleep.
- Don't have a clock within sight.
- Turn off your phone's alerts for texts and emails.
- Write down your worries in a "worry journal." If you can't sleep because you're thinking about something, write it down so you can think about it again the next day.
- If you can't fall asleep after about 20 minutes, get out of bed, and do something relaxing, like reading. When you're ready to sleep again, go back to bed.
- If you want to use your computer late at night, you can get free software for your computer that lets you dim the screen. f.lux and Dimmer are two well-known programs. Even better, turn off the computer an hour before bed.

What to avoid:

- Don't ingest caffeine after noon. This includes soda, coffee, tea, iced tea, and energy drinks.
- Don't drink too much alcohol at night. Alcohol is known to make it easier to fall asleep, but it also makes it harder to stay asleep. This is especially true in the second

half of the night, when the body should be going into deep sleep.

- Don't take other stimulants like chocolate, nicotine, or some medicines close to bedtime.
- Don't eat a big meal right before bed.
- Before bed, don't watch TV, use the computer, or spend a long time on your phone. These things make your brain work, which makes it harder to fall asleep.
- Don't use your phone, laptop, or any other mobile device in bed.
- Don't give in to the urge to take a nap in the middle of the day. It can throw off your normal sleep-wake cycle.

It's essential to note, once again, that you are an individual. You don't necessarily need to follow everything on this list. Some people watch television before bed, and it helps them relax and improves their mood, thus improving their sleep. These recommendations are based on technicalities. Technically, the exposure to the light of the television and the stimulation of what's on screen should have a negative impact on sleep, but if the benefits for you outweigh this minor impact, then sleep can be improved. This applies to almost everything on the list. These should be thought of more as suggestions. Give them a chance and see if they work for you. If something doesn't help or seems to make it worse, stop that. As an extreme example, if drinking a cup of coffee right before bed somehow, paradoxically, helped you sleep, then the fact that nearly everyone on the planet would recommend otherwise is not relevant. Do what works for you. The preceding list is simply a list of methods that have been tested for decades and have been found to work for countless people. They may work for you. They may not.

Histamine

Histamine controls many body functions and is a key part of your body's response to inflammation. Which histamine receptors histamine binds to determines what effect it has. Scientists have found four different kinds of histamine receptors. Excess histamine can cause anxiety as well as insomnia.

H1 receptors

You have H1 receptors all over your body, including in neurons (brain cells), smooth muscle cells in your airways, and blood vessels. When the H1 receptors are turned on, allergy and anaphylaxis symptoms show up. It can lead to:

- Itchy skin (pruritus)
- Anxiety
- Expanding of blood vessels (vasodilation)
- Hypotension (low blood pressure)
- Increased heart rate (tachycardia)
- Flushing
- Narrowing of your airway (bronchoconstriction)
- Pain
- Movement of fluids through blood vessel walls (vascular permeability)
- Some of these changes in the body cause sneezing, stuffy nose, and a runny nose (rhinorrhea).

H1 receptors do more than just control allergic reactions. They also help:

- Sleep-wake cycles
- Food intake
- Body temperature
- Emotions
- Memory
- Learning

Of course, its effect on sleep-wake cycles is our current concern.

Histamine is considered wake-promoting because drowsiness is a common side effect of certain anti-allergy medications that block histamine signaling. Also, histamine neurons are generally active in wake states and inactive during sleep. Histamine neurons promote wakefulness by activating neurons in the cortex that cause arousal and by inhibiting neurons that promote sleep. So, basically, histamine keeps you awake.

How to Reduce Histamine Naturally

Foods that reduce histamine:

- Apples
- Onions
- Pineapple
- Parsley
- Blueberries
- Olive oil
- Vitamin C reduces histamines, as well, so any foods containing vitamin C may reduce histamine.
- Foods to avoid if you trying to reduce histamine:
- Kombucha
- Sauerkraut
- Wine or beer
- Aged meats or cheese
- Olives
- Vinegar
- Canned meats/fish
- Tomatoes
- Ketchup
- Avocados
- Spinach

- Supplements that may help reduce histamine:
- Forskolin
- Quercetin
- Astragalus
- Vitamin C
- B. longum (probiotic strain)
- B. infantis (probiotic strain)
- Erythropoietin
- Pancreatic enzymes (ask a doctor before use)
- Methylxanthines (Dietary sources of methylxanthines include coffee, tea, chocolate, maté, and guarana. You can drink coffee, eat chocolate, or supplement with theobromine, but attempting to supplement with theophylline is not recommended, as adverse cardiac effects are possible. However, chocolate also contains some histamine, and researchers suspect that it may encourage histamine release. The net effect of cocoa is unknown; it's recommended that you test your own individual response and see what it does for you.)
- Fisetin
- Luteolin (found in celery, parsley, and broccoli)
- Apigenin (found in parsley, grapes, and apples)
- EGCG (found in green tea)
- Kaempferol (found in cruciferous vegetables, delphinium plants, witch hazel, and grapefruit)
- Myricetin (found in berries, teas, wines, and many vegetables)
- Rutin (found in buckwheat, apples, and

passionflower)
- Theanine (found in green and black tea)
- Naringenin (found in grapefruit)
- Curcumin (found in turmeric)
- Reishi mushroom
- Chinese Skullcap
- Eleuthero (also known as Siberian ginseng)
- Tulsi (also known as holy basil)
- Mucuna pruriens (also known as velvet bean)
- Vitamin B6
- L. plantarum (a probiotic)
- Palmitoylethanolamide (PEA)
- SAM-e (S-adenosyl-L-methionine)
- Carnosine (made from the amino acids beta-alanine and histidine and found in high-quality meat)
- NAC (N-acetyl cysteine)
- Valine (found in meat, grains, vegetables, and milk and other dairy products)

Drugs that reduce histamine:

- alimemazine (trimeprazine)
- brompheniramine
- chlorphenamine
- dexchlorpheniramine
- diphenhydramine (Benadryl)
- doxylamine (often sold under the brand name "Unisom," though Unisom sometimes contains diphenhydramine instead)
- pheniramine
- promethazine
- triprolidine
- hydroxyzine

These should be reserved for occasional, short-term use

only. You can quickly develop tolerance to them, and side-effects may occur with prolonged use.

Cortisol

Cortisol is a steroid hormone that is made and released by your adrenal glands. These glands are endocrine glands that sit on top of your kidneys. Cortisol affects many parts of your body, but its main job is to control how your body reacts to stress. Cortisol is a hormone called a glucocorticoid that is made and released by your adrenal glands.

Glucocorticoids are a kind of hormone called a steroid. They stop inflammation in your body's tissues and keep your muscles, fat, liver, and bones from breaking down too quickly. Glucocorticoids also change the way people sleep and wake up.

Your body checks your cortisol levels all the time to keep them steady (this is called homeostasis). Cortisol levels that are either too high or too low can be bad for your health.

People often call cortisol the "stress hormone." But it does a lot more than just control your body's stress response. It has many important effects and functions all over your body. Also, it's important to keep in mind that, from a biological point of view, there are many kinds of stress, such as:

Acute stress: This kind of stress happens when you are suddenly and for a short time in danger. Acute stress can be caused by things like barely avoiding a car accident or being chased by an animal.

Chronic stress: This is long-term stress that happens when you must deal with things that make you angry or worried over and over again. Chronic stress can be caused by things like having a job that is hard or frustrating or being sick all the time.

Traumatic stress: This happens when you go through something that puts your life in danger and makes you feel scared and helpless. Traumatic stress can be caused by things like being in a war or being sexually assaulted or going through a tornado. Post-traumatic stress disorder (PTSD) can sometimes be caused by these things.

When any of these things stress you out, your body makes cortisol.

How does my body react to cortisol?

When you're stressed, your body can release cortisol after releasing "fight or flight" hormones like adrenaline. This keeps you on high alert. In times of stress, cortisol also makes your liver release glucose (sugar) so that you can get energy quickly. Cortisol helps control how your body uses fats, proteins, and carbs for energy by regulating your metabolism.

Normally, your cortisol levels are lowest in the evening when you go to sleep and highest in the morning before you wake up. This suggests that cortisol is a key part of waking up and is involved in the circadian rhythm of your body. Cortisol levels need to be just right for people to live and for their bodies to work properly. If your cortisol levels are consistently high or low, it can be bad for your health. High cortisol levels can cause anxiety.

How does my body keep the level of cortisol in check?

Your body has a complicated system to control how much cortisol you have in your body. Your hypothalamus, which is a small part of your brain that controls hormones, and your pituitary gland, which is a small gland below your brain, controls how much cortisol your adrenal glands make. When the amount of cortisol in your blood drops, your hypothalamus releases corticotropin-releasing hormone (CRH), which tells your pituitary gland to make adrenocorticotropic hormone (ACTH). Then, ACTH tells your adrenal glands to make cortisol and let it out. Your hypothalamus, pituitary gland, and adrenal glands must all be working well for you to have the right amount of cortisol in your body.

How can I find out how much cortisol I have?

Your doctor can test your blood, urine, or saliva to see how much cortisol is in your body. Based on your symptoms, they will decide which test is best.

How much cortisol is normal?

Cortisol is a hormone that is found in your blood, urine, and saliva. Its level is highest in the morning and drops throughout the day, reaching its lowest point around midnight. If you work nights and sleep at different times, this pattern can change.

The normal ranges for most tests that measure cortisol in your blood are:

10 to 20 micrograms per deciliter (mcg/dL) from 6 to 8 a.m.

3 to 10 mcg/dL around 4 p.m.

Normal ranges can be different from lab to lab, person to person, and over time. If you need a cortisol level test, your doctor or nurse will look at the results and tell you if you need more testing.

What makes cortisol levels so high?

Hypercortisolism is the medical term for having abnormally high levels of cortisol for a long time. This is usually considered Cushing's Syndrome, which is a rare condition. Causes of cortisol levels that are higher than normal and Cushing's Syndrome include:

Taking a lot of corticosteroid drugs like prednisone, prednisolone, or dexamethasone to treat other health problems.

Tumors that produce adrenocorticotropic hormone (ACTH). These are usually found in your pituitary gland. More rarely, neuroendocrine tumors in other parts of your body such as your lungs can cause high cortisol levels.

Adrenal gland tumors or excessive growth of adrenal tissue (hyperplasia), which cause excess production of cortisol.

What are the signs that your cortisol levels are too high?

Depending on how high your cortisol levels are, your symptoms of Cushing's Syndrome will be different. Common signs and symptoms of cortisol levels that are higher than normal are:

- Weight gain, especially in your face and abdomen.
- Anxiety
- Fatty deposits between your shoulder blades.
- Wide, purple stretch marks on your abdomen (belly).
- Muscle weakness in your upper arms and thighs.
- High blood sugar, which often turns into Type 2 diabetes.
- High blood pressure (hypertension).
- Excessive hair growth (hirsutism) in women.
- Weak bones (osteoporosis) and fractures.

What causes cortisol to be low?

When cortisol levels are lower than normal, this is called hypocortisolism. This is a sign of adrenal insufficiency. There are two kinds of adrenal insufficiency: primary and secondary. Some things that can cause adrenal insufficiency are:

Primary adrenal insufficiency: Most of the time, your immune system attacks healthy cells in your adrenal glands for no known reason, which can cause primary adrenal insufficiency. The name for this is Addison's disease. Your adrenal glands can also be hurt by an infection or bleeding in the tissues (called an adrenal hemorrhage). All these things stop cortisol from being made.

Secondary adrenal insufficiency: If you have hypopituitarism or a tumor on your pituitary gland, it can stop your body from making enough ACTH. ACTH tells your adrenal glands to make cortisol, so when there isn't enough ACTH, there isn't enough cortisol made.

Corticosteroid medications can also cause cortisol levels to be lower than normal, especially if you stop taking them quickly after using them for a long time.

What are the signs that your cortisol levels are too low?

If your cortisol levels are lower than normal, this is called adrenal insufficiency.

- Fatigue
- Anxiety
- Unintentional weight loss
- Poor appetite
- Hypotension (low blood pressure)

How can I lower my level of cortisol?

If you have Cushing's syndrome, which is when your cortisol levels are very high, you will need medical treatment to bring them down. Most treatments involve either medicine or surgery. If your cortisol levels are lower than normal, you'll also need medical help.

In general, though, there are a few simple things you can do every day to try to lower your cortisol levels and keep them where they should be.

Get good sleep: Sleep problems like obstructive sleep apnea, insomnia, or working the night shift can cause cortisol levels to rise.

Regular exercise: Several studies have shown that regular exercise can help you sleep better and feel less stressed, which can lower your cortisol levels over time.

Learn to control stress and stressful ways of thinking: Knowing how you think, how you breathe, how fast your heart beats, and other signs of stress can help you catch it early and stop it from getting worse.

Do exercises that help you take deep breaths: Your parasympathetic nervous system, or "rest and digest" system, is activated when you breathe in a controlled way. This helps lower cortisol levels.

Have fun and laugh: Laughing makes endorphins come out and stops cortisol from coming out. Having hobbies and doing fun things can also make you feel better, which may make your cortisol levels go down.

Keep your relationships in good shape: Relationships are an important part of our life. Having tense, unhealthy relationships with people you care about or work with can cause you to feel stressed out often and raise your cortisol levels.

When should I talk to my doctor about my cortisol levels?

If you have signs of Cushing's syndrome or adrenal insufficiency, you should see a doctor. If you are worried about how stressed you are every day, talk to your doctor or nurse about what you can do to reduce your stress and stay healthy.

Cortisol is a very important hormone that affects a lot of different parts of your body. There are a few things you can do to try to reduce your stress and, by extension, your cortisol levels. However, sometimes you can't help whether your cortisol levels are too high or too low. If you gain or lose weight, or if your blood pressure goes up or down, these are signs that your cortisol levels are too high or too low. You should talk to your doctor about this. They can do some simple tests to find out if your symptoms are caused by your adrenal glands or your pituitary gland.

Foods that lower cortisol:

- Avocados
- Bananas
- Broccoli
- Dark Chocolate
- Seeds
- Spinach
- Nutritional yeast
- Probiotics
- Olive Oil
- Nuts
- Adaptogens such as mushrooms, moringa and ashwagandha
- Cinnamon

Supplements that lower cortisol:

- Ashwagandha
- Omega-3s
- Prebiotics
- Probiotics
- Rhodiola Rosea
- Bacopa Monnieri
- Ginkgo Biloba
- Cordyceps
- Phosphatidylserine
- L-theanine

Norepinephrine

Norepinephrine is a neurotransmitter and a hormone. It is also called noradrenaline. It is a key part of the "fight-or-flight" response in your body. Norepinephrine is also a drug that is used to raise and keep blood pressure high in short-term, serious health situations. As a neurotransmitter, norepinephrine is made from dopamine. Norepinephrine is made by nerve cells in your brainstem and in an area close to your spinal cord. Norepinephrine is a part of your body's sympathetic nervous system, which is part of your "fight-or-flight" response to danger. The "fight or flight" response is called the "acute stress response" in medicine. If you have too much norepinephrine, you may feel anxious or on edge.

How does the body use norepinephrine?

- It makes you more awake, alert, and focused.
- Blood vessels get smaller, which helps keep blood pressure steady when you're stressed.
- Changes the way you sleep, how you feel, and what you remember.

What sets off the release of norepinephrine?

Norepinephrine is a hormone that comes out of your adrenal glands when you're stressed. The fight-or-flight response is the name for the changes in your body that happen because of this response.

What does "fight or flight" mean?

The fight-or-flight response is how your body reacts to stressful situations, like when you need to get away from a dangerous situation (like a dog that is growling) or when you have to face a fear (like giving a speech for school or work). During the fight-or-flight response, your brain tells you that something bad is happening. Then, nerves in a part of your brain called the hypothalamus send a message down your spinal cord and out to the rest of your body. Norepinephrine is the neurotransmitter that tells your nervous system what to do when your brain tells it what to do. The neurotransmitter noradrenaline goes to these organs and tissues and causes these quick reactions in the body:

Eyes: The pupils get bigger to let in more light so you can see more of what's around you.

Skin: Your skin goes pale when your blood vessels get a message to send blood to places that need it more, like your muscles, so you can fight or run away.

Heart: The heart beats harder and faster to get more oxygenated blood to places like your muscles that need it most. Also, blood pressure goes up.

Muscles: When muscles get more blood flow and oxygen, they can move and work faster and with more strength.

Liver: Your liver turns the glycogen you have stored into glucose, which gives you more energy.

Airways: People breathe faster and deeper. Your airways widen, which lets more oxygen into your blood, which then goes to your muscles.

Your adrenal gland releases the hormones adrenaline (epinephrine) and noradrenaline (norepinephrine) when the neurotransmitter noradrenaline gets to it. These hormones get to every part of your body through your blood. They go back to your eyes, heart, lungs, skin, blood vessels, and adrenal gland. The "message" to these organs and tissues is to keep reacting until the danger is gone.

Norepinephrine is used as a medicine to raise and keep blood pressure up in situations where low blood pressure is a problem, but only for a short time. Some of these conditions could be:

- Cardiac arrest
- Spinal anesthesia
- Septicemia
- Blood transfusions
- Drug reactions

Low levels of norepinephrine can cause the following

health problems:

- Anxiety
- Depression
- ADHD
- Headache
- Memory problems
- Sleeping problems
- Hypotension (low blood pressure)
- Low blood sugar (hypoglycemia)
- Blood pressure and heart rate changes
- Dopamine beta-hydroxylase deficiency. Your body can't turn dopamine into norepinephrine if you have this rare genetic disease

High levels of epinephrine can cause the following health problems:

- High blood pressure
- Rapid or irregular heartbeat
- Excessive sweating
- Pale or cold skin
- Frequent headaches
- Nervous feeling, jitters
- Pheochromocytoma, which is a growth on the adrenal glands

People with high levels of norepinephrine are more likely to hurt their heart, blood vessels, or kidneys. To lower norepinephrine, it's important to find ways to put your body into parasympathetic response mode, so anything in nature that can help you relax will do. Norepinephrine levels can be kept in check by eating a well-balanced diet, reducing emotional and physical stress, getting enough sleep, and exercising regularly.

Nutrition

A well-balanced diet has been shown to help keep your

immune system healthy and give you the extra energy you need to deal with stress. Early research suggests that omega-3 fatty acids and vegetables may help control cortisol levels. Mindful eating reduces stress by encouraging people to take deep breaths, choose their food carefully, pay attention to the meal, and chew their food slowly and thoroughly. This can also help your body digest better.

Herbs and Supplements

Calming amino acids like a theanine supplement can help support norepinephrine levels, and nervine botanicals like lemon balm, kava, and chamomile, which work on the nervous system, can help naturally lower norepinephrine levels.

There has been a lot of research on how adaptogenic herbs like ashwagandha can help the nervous system adapt to stressors, which can reduce stress and anxiety in people who use them regularly.

Melatonin has been shown to lower the amount of norepinephrine in the body because it helps the sympathetic tone.

Lifestyle

Physical activity can help lower stress hormones and blood pressure. Aerobic exercise raises your heart rate and breathing rate, which lets more oxygen flow through your body.

Meditation, yoga, and tai chi all focus on deep breathing, which can help the parasympathetic nervous system help fight stress.

Some research shows that using cognitive behavioral therapy (CBT) can help lower norepinephrine levels, which are often high in people who are anxious or angry.

Supplements

Many supplements are known to assist sleep. Here are some of the better known and more widely used and studied ones available.

Lavender

Lavender oil seems to have a soothing effect and reduces anxiety and restlessness. Most studies on lavender's efficacy as a sleep aid have focused on lavender essential oil, though some people also use the dried herb as a tea or in their pillow. Essential oils should not be ingested except under a doctor's supervision, as even lavender oil contains poisonous compounds. Instead, the oil should be diffused into the air or diluted in a neutral cream or oil for use on the skin.

Lavender may be most appealing for people who struggle to sleep due to anxiety or racing thoughts. It is also popular among people who want an external sleep aid rather than something they consume. Short-term use of dried lavender or use of lavender essential oil is thought to be safe, though potential side effects for the external use of lavender oil include skin irritation and allergic reaction.

Lavendar is also available as a clinically-studied supplement called Lavela WS 1265.

Valerian

Valerian has been used for sleep problems since the 2nd century. Though further research needs to be done, valerian appears to help people fall asleep faster, sleep better, and wake up less often. In some studies, patients taking valerian were 80% more likely to report sleep improvements than those taking a placebo.

Because experts have not located a single active compound, they speculate that valerian's effect may be due to several compounds working together, or the amino acids GABA or glycine.

The roots and stems of the valerian plant are made into teas, tinctures, capsules, extracts, and tablets. While each type of preparation has its fans, the tea can have an unpleasant odor, and researchers generally use liquid extracts or capsules in their research. Valerian is usually recommended for people with insomnia or general problems with sleep quality. Most people report that it is more effective once they have been taking it for several weeks. However, further research is needed to determine how effective valerian is in treating insomnia.

Valerian is generally considered safe for adults. Side effects are rare and tend to be mild but may include headache, dizziness, itching, and upset stomach.

German Chamomile

German chamomile has been used to treat sleep problems since ancient Egypt. Despite this long history, there has been little research into its benefits. What we do know from smaller studies and meta-analysis is that German chamomile may soothe anxiety and improve sleep quality, although researchers are not clear on why it might have these effects. On the other hand, it does not appear to benefit people with insomnia.

The most common preparations of German chamomile are capsules, tincture, and tea. Although there is another variety called Roman chamomile, most research has focused on the German type.

Chamomile is generally regarded as safe when used as a tea or taken orally. It does have potential interactions with some drugs, including blood thinners, and there is little information on its safety for those who are pregnant or breastfeeding. Side effects are usually limited to mild nausea or dizziness, but allergic reactions are possible, particularly for people with allergies to related plants like ragweed and daisies.

Passionflower

The passionflower vine is native to the Americas and has historically been used as a sedative by multiple indigenous cultures. There has been very little research into its benefits, though the existing research is encouraging, if limited. In one study focused on generalized anxiety disorder, passionflower's calming effects were comparable to a commonly prescribed sedative. Passionflower may also improve sleep quality and make it easier to fall and stay asleep.

Extracts and tea are both common forms of passionflower people use. Both have been used in research settings, so choosing between them is a matter of preference. While research into this supplement shows potential benefits for anxiety and insomnia, there is no conclusive proof of its efficacy.

There is little research into its safety. However, daily doses of up to 800 milligrams have been used safely in studies lasting as long as two months. Side effects are usually mild and may include drowsiness, confusion, and uncoordinated movements. Pregnant women should not use passionflower, as it can induce uterine contractions. There is limited research into its safety while breastfeeding.

Hops

In addition to being the main flavoring in beer, the flowers of the hops plant are used by some people as a natural sleep aid. Like most natural supplements, the benefits of hops have not been researched enough to definitively state whether it might help people sleep better. However, there is preliminary evidence that hops supplements can help stabilize circadian rhythms and lessen the symptoms of shift work disorder. Dried hops flowers contain the acids humulone and lupulone, and their relationship with the body's GABA receptors may be part of the reason for hops' effects.

Hops is often combined with other natural sleep aids such as valerian. It can be taken as non-alcoholic beer or in dried form as a tea or dry extract. Different studies have used all three methods, and there is no evidence in favor of one form over another.

It is likely safe to consume hops in the form of non-alcoholic beer or tea, though supplemental use is only considered possibly safe due to the lack of research. Hops also has more potential side effects than some other natural sleep aids. Because it has weak effects similar to estrogen, hops can cause changes to the menstrual cycle and is not recommended for people who are pregnant or breastfeeding, or who have hormone-sensitive cancers or other conditions. Hops can also worsen depression. However, for most people, side effects are mild and may include dizziness or sleepiness.

Cannabidiol (CBD)

CBD is a chemical known as a cannabinoid that is present in the cannabis plant. Cannabis has over 100 cannabinoids, and CBD is much different than the psychoactive delta-9-tetrahydrocannabinol (THC) cannabinoid. Most CBD is derived from hemp, which does not contain enough THC to be psychoactive.

Research into CBD has previously been limited due to cannabis regulations, but there are indications that it might help some people sleep better. To begin with, it appears to reduce the anxious symptoms of a broad spectrum of mental health conditions. It also seems that the body's own cannabinoid system affects how we sleep, making CBD more likely to have benefits. There has been some evidence that CBD can aid some sleep disorders and reduce excessive daytime sleepiness, but research is currently inconclusive.

Although CBD has been legal federally since 2018, it is not supposed to be sold as a dietary supplement. It is, however, widely available in forms such as tinctures, gummies, and oils. Because of this lack of regulatory oversight, one study found that 26% of CBD products had less CBD than they claimed, while 43% had much more. CBD appears to be largely safe with minor side effects such as tiredness, diarrhea, and changes to weight or appetite. However, its safety is unknown for people who are pregnant or breastfeeding CBD may interact with medications and adversely impact certain health conditions.

Tart Cherry Juice

Juice from the tart cherry, also known as the sour cherry, appears to raise melatonin levels and increase the availability of tryptophan, an amino acid that may play a role in helping people fall asleep. These are promising findings, and tart cherry juice may improve sleep quality and make it easier to fall asleep. However, some studies indicate that the effect on insomnia is not as strong as established treatments like cognitive-behavioral therapy.

Studies on the health benefits of tart cherries have had participants consume the equivalent of up to 270 cherries a day, but there is no specific research into their safety. The juice, which can be very sour, is usually diluted in a small amount of water before drinking.

Magnesium

Magnesium is a mineral naturally present in food and often added to processed foods. It is used throughout the body and is present in bones, soft tissue, and blood. Older adults are more at risk for magnesium deficiency, and one of the mineral's many roles is sleep regulation. Some research suggests that supplemental magnesium may help reduce insomnia in older adults, either when used alone or with melatonin and zinc. It may also reduce excessive daytime sleepiness in adults.

Since high levels of magnesium are available in foods like pumpkin seeds, it is easy to supplement by eating more magnesium-rich foods. Magnesium supplements are also available in pills and tablets, including multivitamins. Magnesium aspartate, magnesium citrate, magnesium lactate, and magnesium chloride are the easiest for the body to absorb.

While magnesium is usually safe at ordinary dietary levels since the kidneys filter it out, high dosages can cause side effects like diarrhea, nausea, and abdominal cramping. Magnesium also interacts with some medication and other supplements, and very large dosages can lead to significant heart abnormalities including low blood pressure or hypotension, irregular heartbeat, and cardiac arrest.

GABA

Gamma-aminobutyric acid (GABA) is an amino acid and neurotransmitter that plays a vital role in regulating nervous system activity. In addition to being made by the body and present in food like tea and tomatoes, GABA is available in supplement form. While it was previously believed that GABA taken orally could not pass the blood-brain barrier and was therefore not useful to the body, there is now some evidence to the contrary

Small trials of supplemental GABA have shown that it can reduce stress and may help people fall asleep more easily. It is not currently known whether GABA's effects on sleep might be due to stress reduction or another mechanism.

GABA naturally occurs in the body and in food, but there is little research into whether it is safe to take as a supplement. However, most studies have shown no adverse reactions. GABA is available in pills and may be derived from natural or synthetic sources. Research is still ongoing as to whether synthetic GABA is as effective as GABA derived from a natural source.

Glycine

Like GABA, glycine is an amino acid and neurotransmitter made by the body and available in some foods. Glycine appears to affect sleep and pass the blood-brain barrier. Studies show that glycine appears to improve sleep quality, potentially by lowering body temperature. Taking glycine before bed may also help reduce the negative effects of insufficient sleep, which may be due to improved sleep quality or another mechanism.

Supplemental glycine is available in capsule or powder

form, and there is limited knowledge about what form might be most beneficial. While glycine is part of our diet, its safety is unknown when taken in the quantities usually found in supplements.

Are Natural Sleep Aids Safe?

Natural sleep aids are not universally safe or unsafe. Sold over the counter or online, natural sleep aids do not go through the same testing and review process as prescription medicines.

In general, there is a lack of high-quality research about the effectiveness and safety of most natural sleep aids. As a result, many questions about natural sleep remedies remain unresolved. There are special considerations to keep in mind when evaluating the safety of natural sleep aids.

Adults

Many natural sleep remedies, when taken in the proper dosage by healthy adults, have few side effects. But this does not mean that all natural sleep aids are safe.

As a precaution, adults should talk with their doctor or pharmacist before taking a natural sleep aid. Adults should also stop taking natural sleep aids if they notice any abnormal health changes or side effects.

Children

Some natural sleep aids may be safe for use in children, though sleep hygiene should be encouraged before sleep aids are considered. In many cases, there is insufficient research in children to confidently evaluate the safety or efficacy of natural sleep aids.

For certain natural sleep aids, such as melatonin, short-term use is generally considered to be safe for most children, but there is limited data about long-term use.

To make sure that any medication or sleep aid does not affect their child's health and development, parents should take precautions when considering natural sleep aids for their children, including:

Talking with their pediatrician first

Ensuring that the dosage is meant for children and not adults

Paying attention to the label and list of ingredients

Looking for high-quality products that are tested by third parties to reduce the risk of tainted or mislabeled supplements

Pregnant or Breastfeeding

People who are pregnant or breastfeeding should use caution with natural sleep aids. Many ingredients have not gone through rigorous testing in people who are pregnant or breastfeeding, so little is known about potential effects on their child.

Although some products may be safe, the best approach for those who are pregnant or breastfeeding is to consult with their doctor prior to taking natural sleep aids.

Should You Talk to a Doctor Before Taking a Natural Sleep Aid?

It is advisable to talk with a doctor before starting to use any natural sleep aid. Even though these products are available without a prescription, your doctor may be able to help in several ways:

Reviewing your other medications and the potential for interactions between them and a natural sleep aid

Addressing your health history and the likelihood of adverse reactions from natural sleep aids

Understanding your sleeping problems and evaluating if they may be caused by an underlying sleep disorder that can be resolved with a more specific form of treatment

Discussing the potential benefits and risks of specific types of natural sleep aids

Offering suggestions about dosage or timing for taking natural sleep aids

Providing guidance about how to know whether a natural sleep aid is working or causing side-effects

Cognitive Behavioral Therapy for Insomnia (CBT-I)

Cognitive behavioral therapy for insomnia (CBT-I or CBTI) is a short, structured, and evidence-based way to deal with the frustrating symptoms of insomnia.

How it Works

CBT-I tries to figure out how the way we think, what we do, and how we sleep are all linked. During treatment, a trained CBT-I provider helps figure out what thoughts, feelings, and actions are causing the insomnia symptoms.

Thoughts and feelings about sleep are looked at and tested to see if they are true. Behaviors are also looked at to see if they help people get to sleep. Then, a provider will clear up or reframe any misunderstandings or problems in a way that makes it easier to sleep.

Most treatments take between 6 and 8 sessions. The length can vary depending on what a person needs. When given by a primary care doctor, treatment can be as short as two visits.

People often call CBT-I a "multicomponent treatment" because it uses more than one method. Sessions can have educational, cognitive, and behavioral parts.

Cognitive interventions include "cognitive restructuring," which tries to change wrong or harmful ideas about sleep.

Behavior changes can include relaxation training,

controlling stimuli, and limiting sleep. All these help people relax and get into good sleep habits.

At the heart of CBT-I is giving information about how thoughts, feelings, behaviors, and sleep are connected. The order and flow of each part can change based on how the provider works and what each person needs. Here are some CBT-I techniques that are often used:

Cognitive Restructuring

People with insomnia may have wrong or dysfunctional thoughts about sleep, which can make them do things that make it harder to sleep. This reinforces the wrong or dysfunctional thoughts.

For example, having trouble sleeping before can make it hard to fall asleep again. This worry might make you stay in bed for too long to try to sleep. Both stress and spending too much time in bed can make it harder to fall asleep and stay asleep. This can turn into a frustrating nightly pattern that can be hard to break.

Cognitive restructuring starts to break this cycle by identifying, challenging, and changing the thoughts and beliefs that lead to insomnia. During treatment, common thoughts and beliefs that may be addressed include anxiety about past episodes of insomnia, having unrealistic expectations about sleep time and quality, and worrying about being tired during the day or other effects of not getting enough sleep.

With the help of a trained provider who can help evaluate them more objectively, inaccurate thoughts can be found, challenged, and changed. Homework is often given so that students can practice these skills when they are not in class.

Stimulus Control

People who can't sleep start to dread going to bed because they associate it with being awake and frustrated. They may also think of their bedroom as a place where they do things that make it hard to sleep, like eat, watch TV, or use a cell phone or computer. Stimulus control tries to change how these things are linked.

During treatment, the bed is only used for sleeping and making love. Clients are told to get out of bed if they can't fall asleep or if they've been awake for more than 10 minutes. They should only go back to bed when they're tired again. Clients are told to set their alarms for the same time every morning and not to nap during the day.

Sleep Restriction and Compression

People with insomnia often lie awake in bed for too long. Sleep restriction limits how long a person can stay in bed so that they can get back on a regular sleep schedule.

This technique is meant to make you want to sleep more and can temporarily make you feel more tired during the day. It is not recommended for people with health problems like bipolar disorder and seizures that can get worse when they don't get enough sleep.

Using a sleep diary, the first step in sleep restriction is to figure out how long a typical night of sleep is. The amount of time in bed is then changed by this amount plus 30 minutes. For example, if a person wants to sleep 8 hours a night but only gets 5, they should change their bedtime so that they sleep for 5 hours and 30 minutes. Once a person spends most of their time in bed sleeping, they can start slowly extending the amount of time they spend there.

Sleep compression is a slightly different method that is often used with older people because it is gentler. Instead of immediately cutting down the amount of time they spend in bed to the amount of sleep they get on an average night, the time they spend in bed is gradually cut down until it is close to the amount of time they spend sleeping.

Relaxation Training

Relaxation techniques can help ease the stress and racing thoughts that come with lying awake in bed. These methods can boost the body's natural ability to calm down. This is good for both the body and the mind.

The best ways to relax are those that are easy to fit into a person's daily life. Here are a few CBT-I techniques that are often used to help people relax:

Breathing exercises: CBT-I can teach many different breathing exercises. Most of these exercises have you take slow, deep breaths. Research has shown that focused breathing can slow down your heart rate and breathing, as well as make you feel less anxious, angry, and sad.

Progressive Muscle Relaxation (PMR): PMR is a method in which different muscle groups are tense and then relaxed. These techniques can be used with guided imagery or breathing exercises.

Autogenic training is a way to focus on different parts of the body and pay attention to certain feelings. A person can pay attention to feelings like weight, warmth, or relaxation.

Biofeedback is a technique that uses technology to help keep track of things like brain waves, heart rate, breathing, and body temperature. People may be able to learn to have more control over these processes if they use the information that electronic devices give them.

Guided or self-hypnosis can help people who have trouble sleeping by teaching them how to relax when given a verbal or non-verbal cue.

Meditation has many benefits, such as lowering stress and anxiety and making it easier to relax. Meditation can also be done through practices like yoga and tai chi that combine focused attention with movement.

Psychoeducation

A core part of CBT-I is teaching clients how important good sleep hygiene is. Good sleep hygiene means doing more things that help you sleep and lessening or getting rid of things that make it hard to sleep.

Some of the things that might be talked about are how diet, exercise, and the place you sleep affect your ability to fall asleep and stay asleep.

Homework

CBT-I is a group process, and practicing the skills you learn in sessions is important. A common part of treatment is giving the patient homework. Between sessions, you might have to do things like keep a sleep diary, practice questioning automatic thoughts or beliefs when they come up and improve your sleep hygiene.

Is CBT-I helpful?

When these techniques are used together as part of CBT-I with multiple components, between 70% and 80% of people with primary insomnia feel better. It takes less time to fall asleep, you sleep longer, and you wake up less often during sleep. Results tend to stay the same over time.

For some people, CBT-I works better than medications. This treatment has also been shown to work for people who are more likely than others to have trouble sleeping, such as pregnant women.

CBT-I is thought to help with many kinds of insomnia. It may even help people with short-term insomnia. This means that CBT-I may be useful for treating insomnia symptoms even if they don't meet the criteria for chronic insomnia.

Even though this treatment for insomnia has been shown to be very effective, it doesn't always work right away. It can take time to learn and use the skills that are taught in therapy. Some methods, like controlling what you do before bed and getting less sleep, can help you change your sleep habits slowly. Some people find it helpful to keep track of their progress over time so they can see small improvements that can encourage them to keep going with treatment.

If CBT-I alone doesn't help with insomnia symptoms, the American College of Physicians suggests talking to a doctor about the risks and benefits of taking sleep medications along with CBT-I.

Does CBT-I Have Risks?

For CBT-I to work, you need to be willing to face your negative thoughts and actions. Even though the risks of treatment are likely to be low, it may sometimes be painful. Talking about painful memories, thoughts, and feelings can be hard and may cause stress and discomfort in the short term.

Working with a trained CBT-I professional can help reduce the risks of this treatment because they know how to give support and tools to deal with temporary problems or setbacks.

Who Gives CBT-I?

CBT-I is usually given by a doctor, counselor, therapist, or psychiatrist who has been trained to do so. Professional groups like the Society of Behavioral Sleep Medicine and the American Board of Sleep Medicine can help you find CBT-I practitioners.

There aren't enough CBT-I professionals to meet the demand right now because so many people need this treatment. Researchers have come up with new ways to offer CBT-I, like digital, group, and self-help formats.

Digital CBT-I

Several digital CBT-I (sometimes called dCBT-I or dCBT) apps have been made to keep up with this trend, lower the cost of treatment, and give more people access to the benefits of CBT-I. The Department of Veterans Affairs has its own app called CBT-I Coach. It can be used by both veterans and people who are not veterans.

Different online resources and smartphone apps that offer dCBT-I have different purposes and require different amounts of help from the provider. Some resources just help people while they work with a trained CBT-I provider in person, while others are fully automated and don't need any help from a clinician. Other resources and apps are a mix of the two, letting people work through a pre-set program and have regular feedback sessions with a professional through e-mail or the phone.

Digital CBT-I works well to treat insomnia in kids, teens, and adults.

Even though only a few studies have directly compared dCBT-I and face-to-face approaches, it seems that both help people with insomnia feel better.

Medication

In some cases, doctors will prescribe drugs for the treatment of insomnia. All insomnia medications should be taken shortly before bed. Do not attempt to drive or perform other activities that require concentration after taking an insomnia drug because it will make you sleepy and can increase your risk for accidents. Medications should be used in combination with good sleep practices. Here are some medications that can be used to treat insomnia:

Antidepressants

Some antidepressant drugs, such as trazodone (Desyrel), are very good at treating sleeplessness and anxiety.

Benzodiazepines

These older sleeping pills -- emazepam (Restoril), triazolam (Halcion), and others -- may be useful when you want an insomnia medication that stays in the system longer. For instance, they have been effectively used to treat sleep problems such as sleepwalking and night terrors. These medications have some serious downsides. They can cause addiction and dependence. Dependence means that you have physical withdrawal when you stop them. Also, there is a black box warning against their use with opioids, because both depress respiration and increase your risk of overdose.

Doxepine (Silenor)

This sleep drug is approved for use in people who have trouble staying asleep. Silenor may help with sleep maintenance by blocking histamine receptors. Do not take this drug unless you have time to get a full 7 or 8 hours of sleep.

Eszopiclone (Lunesta)

Lunesta also helps you fall asleep quickly, and studies show people sleep an average of 7 to 8 hours while on it. Don't take Lunesta unless you are able to get a full night's sleep as it could cause grogginess. Because of the risk of impairment the next day, the FDA recommends the starting dose of Lunesta be no more than 1 milligram.

Lemborexant (Dayvigo)

This drug is approved for people who have trouble falling asleep and staying asleep. It works by suppressing the part of the central nervous system that keeps you awake. It may cause you to feel sleepy the next day.

Ramelteon (Rozerem)

This sleep medication works differently than the others. It works by targeting the sleep-wake cycle, not by depressing the central nervous system. It is prescribed for people who have trouble falling asleep. Rozerem can be prescribed for long-term use, and the drug has shown no evidence of abuse or dependence.

Suvorexant (Belsomra)

It works by blocking a hormone that promotes wakefulness and causes insomnia. It is approved by the FDA to treat people that have insomnia due to an inability to fall asleep or to stay asleep. The drug may cause you to feel sleepy the following day.

Zaleplon (Sonata)

Of all the newer sleeping pills, Sonata stays active in the body for the shortest amount of time. That means you can try to fall asleep on your own, then, if you're still staring at the clock at 2 a.m., you can take it without feeling drowsy in the morning. But if you tend to wake during the night, this might not be the best choice for you.

Zolpidem (Ambien, Edluar, Intermezzo)

These medicines work well at helping you get to sleep, but some people tend to wake up in the middle of the night. Zolpidem is now available in an extended-release version, Ambien CR. This may help you go to sleep and stay asleep longer. The FDA warns that you should not drive or do anything that requires you to be alert the day after taking Ambien CR because it stays in the body a long time. You should not take zolpidem unless you are able to get a full night's sleep -- at least 7 to 8 hours. In rare instances, these medications have been known to cause injuries because of behaviors while asleep or partially asleep such as sleep walking and sleep driving, among others. The FDA has approved a prescription oral spray called Zolpimist, which contains zolpidem, for the short-term treatment of insomnia brought on by trouble falling asleep.

If these medications don't work for you, your doctor may suggest something off-label. These are medications used to treat conditions they weren't originally made for. Older antidepressants are sometimes prescribed to treat insomnia because they change brain chemicals, which can help regulate sleep. These older medications also tend to have a sedative effect or make you sleepy.

They include:

- Amitriptyline (Elavil)
- Mirtazapine (Remeron SolTab, Remeron)
- Nortriptyline (Aventyl, Pamelor)
- Trazodone
- Gabapentin
- Tiagabine

The FDA issued warnings for prescription sleep drugs, alerting patients that they can cause rare allergic reactions and complex sleep-related behaviors, including "sleep driving." They also warned people that taking sleeping medication at night can impair their ability to drive or be fully alert -- even the next day.

Keep in mind that sleep drugs are not for long-term use. Talk to your doctor if you're still having trouble sleeping after 2 weeks. For a short time, a sleeping pill can help you sleep better. But it's important to know everything about sleeping pills that you need to know. That means knowing about the side effects of sleeping pills. If you do, you can avoid using these sleep aids in the wrong way.

What are sleeping pills?

The name for most sleeping pills is "sedative hypnotics." That's a group of drugs that help people fall asleep or stay asleep. Benzodiazepines, barbiturates, and other hypnotics are examples of sedative hypnotics.

Anti-anxiety drugs like Ativan, Librium, Valium, and Xanax are called benzodiazepines. They also make people feel sleepy and help them fall asleep. Halcion is an older sedative-hypnotic benzodiazepine drug that has been mostly replaced by newer drugs. Even though these drugs may help in the short term, all benzodiazepines have the potential to become addicting and can make it hard to remember things and pay attention. Most of the time, they are not recommended as a long-term solution for trouble sleeping.

Barbiturates are another type of sedative-hypnotic drug. They slow down the central nervous system and can make you sleepy. As sedatives or sleeping pills, barbiturates can have a short or long effect. Most of the time, though, these drugs are only used as anesthesia. If you take too much, they can kill you.

Newer drugs help you fall asleep more quickly. Ambien, Lunesta, and Sonata are all sleep-inducing drugs that bind to the same brain receptors as benzodiazepines. They are less likely to cause physical dependence than benzodiazepines, but they can still sometimes do so over time. They can work quickly to make you feel sleepy and help you fall asleep. Rozerem is a different kind of sleep aid from the ones we've already talked about. It changes melatonin, a hormone in the brain, and it's not addictive. Belsomra is a unique sleep aid that works on a chemical in the brain called orexin. It is not addictive. Silenor, a low-dose version of the tricyclic antidepressant doxepin, is another non-addictive sleep aid.

What do sleeping pills do to your body?

Like most medicines, sleeping pills can make you feel bad in other ways. But you won't know if a certain sleeping pill will cause side effects until you try it.

If you have asthma or other health problems, your doctor may be able to tell you about some side effects. Sleeping pills can make it hard to breathe normally and can be dangerous for people with asthma, emphysema, or some types of chronic obstructive pulmonary disease (COPD), which is a lung disease that makes it hard to breathe.

Sleeping pills like Ambien, Halcion, Lunesta, Rozerem, and Sonata often have the following side effects:

- Hands, arms, feet, or legs that burn or tingle
- Changes in appetite
- Constipation
- Diarrhea
- Balance problems
- Dizziness
- Day-time drowsiness
- Dry throat or mouth
- Gas
- Headache
- Heartburn
- Impairment the following day
- Slowing of the mind or trouble paying attention or remembering
- Pain or tenderness in the stomach
- Shaking of a body part that can't be stopped
- Unusual dreams
- Weakness

It's important to know about the possible side effects of sleeping pills so you can stop taking them and call your doctor right away if you start to feel sick.

Sleeping Pills and Older Adults

Experts say you shouldn't use any sleep aids if you're 65 or older. This includes both over-the-counter drugs and newer "Z" drugs like eszopiclone (Lunesta), zaleplon (Sonata), and zolpidem (Ambien).

When taking sleep aids, older adults are more likely to get sick than younger people. When you're older, sleeping pills tend to stay in your system longer. After taking them, you might feel sleepy all day. Confusion and trouble remembering things are also known to happen. This could cause older people to trip and fall, break their hips, or get into car accidents.

Some over-the-counter sleep aids can cause other side effects that are hard for older people to deal with. You might have a dry mouth. You could also be constipated and have trouble going to the bathroom.

Before you decide to take sleeping pills, talk to your doctor. They may suggest that you get a medical exam to find out what's causing your sleep problems, such as depression, anxiety, or a sleep disorder. Your doctor will also give you ideas for how to treat your inability to sleep without drugs.

Are there sleep-aid side effects that are more complicated?

Some sleeping pills have side effects that could be harmful, such as parasomnia. Parasomnias are movements, behaviors, and actions like sleepwalking that you can't stop. During a parasomnia, you're asleep and don't know what's going on around you.

Parasomnias are complicated sleep behaviors that can happen when you take sleeping pills. For example, you might eat, talk on the phone, or have sex while you're sleeping. Another bad side effect of sleeping pills is sleep driving, which is driving while not fully awake. Even though parasomnias are rare, they are hard to notice once the medicine starts to work.

On the labels of sleep aids and hypnotics, there is information about the possible risks of taking a sleeping pill. Because complex sleep behaviors are more likely to happen if you take more than what your doctor tells you to, don't take more than what your doctor tells you to.

Can I have an allergic reaction to sleep aids?

Yes. People can be allergic to any medicine. The allergy could be caused by the medicine's active ingredient or by one of its inactive ingredients, like dyes, binders, or coatings. People who are allergic to a certain sleeping pill should stay away from it. At the first sign of any of these serious side effects, you should talk to your doctor right away:

- Blurry vision or any other eye problems
- Chest pain
- Difficulty breathing or swallowing
- Feeling like your throat is closing
- Hives
- Hoarseness
- Itching
- Nausea
- Rapidly beating heart
- Rash
- Eye, face, lip, tongue, or throat swelling
- Vomiting

Also, anaphylaxis is a serious side effect that can even kill someone who is allergic to a medicine. Anaphylaxis is a sudden reaction to an allergy. Angioedema, which is a severe swelling of the face, is another possible side effect. Again, if you are allergic, you should talk to your doctor about these possibilities.

When do I take a pill to help me sleep?

Most of the time, it's best to take a sleeping pill right before you want to go to bed. Read the instructions your doctor wrote on the label of the sleeping pill. There is specific information about your medicine in the directions. Also, always give yourself enough time to sleep before taking a sleeping pill.

TENS (Transcutaneous Electrical Nerve Stimulation)

TENS Units, which use electrical stimulation, are the least talked about way to help people sleep, anxiety, and other mental health concerns. In one study, people with chronic insomnia took part in an open trial to see how well low frequency electrical stimulation helped them sleep. Fifty-four people were studied for four weeks. A TENS Unit was put on their trapezius muscle five days a week, 30 minutes to an hour before bed. The study's results showed that low-frequency electrical stimulation made poor sleep and insomnia a lot easier to deal with. This also made people feel less sleepy during the day, which helped improve their overall quality of life.

There are many high-quality TENS machines available online. Some of the best options are made by Oxiline.

EMS (Electrical Muscle Stimulation)

Electrical muscle stimulation (EMS) technology supports muscle recovery and helps reduce tension and muscle discomfort, thereby supporting better sleep. From professional athletes and fitness enthusiasts to busy moms and everyday people who experience muscle pain or muscle atrophy, electric muscle stimulation offers a safe, scientifically sound way to support fitness recovery, decrease muscle pain and enhance a healthy sleep schedule.

EMS devices typically come with a dual function which includes TENS. There are many viable options, but for a wide variety of choices, you can check out Therabody.

Acupuncture

There are many reports that acupuncture helps a lot with insomnia with very few side-effects, but there has yet to be a systematic study of its efficacy and safety.

Hypnosis

People often get the wrong idea about hypnosis because of how it is shown in movies and TV shows. Because of this, it is often overlooked or written off as a possible treatment for a wide range of health problems. When done in a specific way, hypnosis can help a person pay attention in a way that makes it easier for them to listen to suggestions that can help them change the way they think and act. Early research shows that it may help people with insomnia and other sleep problems and has few side effects.

Before starting sleep hypnosis, it's important to know what it is, how it works, what its pros and cons are, and how to get the most out of it.

Hypnosis is a state of mind where a person is very focused on a single thought or image. This makes them less aware of their surroundings and can make them seem to be in a trance-like state. During hypnosis, the brain activity of a person changes, making them more open to new ideas.

Hypnotherapy has been shown to help with pain and some side effects of cancer treatment, among other health problems. It can help with some mental health problems.

Hypnosis does not control the mind. During hypnosis, a person is usually more receptive to suggestions, but they still have control over what they do. Most worries about mind control come from stage shows or TV shows that don't show how hypnosis is used in real medicine. Even though some people who are very easy to hypnotize may seem to be completely controlled by a hypnotist, decades of research show that hypnosis is not the same as mind control.

Hypnosis does not involve falling asleep. Instead, a person stays awake, but their attention is fixed in a way that might make them look like they are in a trance or just not paying attention.

Sleep hypnosis is when hypnotherapy is used to help people who have trouble sleeping. Sleep hypnosis is not meant to make someone fall asleep during the hypnosis. Instead, it changes bad sleep-related thoughts or habits so that the person can sleep better after hypnotherapy.

Hypnosis can help people sleep, but it can be used with other treatments as well. For instance, it can be used with cognitive behavioral therapy for insomnia (CBT-I).. Sleep hypnosis may also help people develop better sleep habits and better sleep hygiene.

Aromatherapy

Essential oils are oils derived from plants, usually by crushing and steam distilling parts of the plant. A variety of essential oils have been used as medical treatments since ancient times. Aromatherapy involves inhaling essential oil scents or vapor in hopes of obtaining positive health effects. Research demonstrates that because smell affects sleep, incorporating certain essential oils into your bedtime routine may help people sleep better.

Learn about the best essential oils for sleep to determine which ones you want to bring into your bedroom environment.

.Lavender

Lavender, a purple flowering shrub, seems to be the plant with the essential oil that is most studied by scientists. This essential oil calms the nervous system, primarily due to the chemical compounds linalool and linalyl acetate found within it. Many studies demonstrate lavender's positive effect on sleep in a variety of people.

People with insomnia — especially women, younger people, and those with mild insomnia — reported improved sleep after breathing in steam filled with lavender essential oil. In students, exposure to lavender aroma at nighttime reduced sleepiness upon waking the following day. Ischemic heart disease patients sleeping in a hospital's intensive care unit experienced improved quality of sleep after hours of lavender aromatherapy. Women between ages 45 and 55 experienced improved sleep quality after lavender aromatherapy. Hospital patients with coronary artery disease experienced improved sleep and reduced anxiety after inhaling a lavender essential oil. Postpartum mothers who inhaled lavender essential oil and kept cotton balls soaked with lavender essential oil in the room as they slept enjoyed improved sleep.

Lavender can be put on a pillow to be inhaled during the night or combined with other oils and used for massage, as it is easily absorbed by the skin. Combining lavender aromatherapy with sleep hygiene techniques improves sleep more than lavender alone.

Bergamot

Bergamot is a fragrant herb native to North America, often grown to attract pollinators such as bees and butterflies. Research suggests bergamot may help with a variety of ailments. Sometimes, bergamot is ingested in extract form or as a juice. Bergamot essential oil may also be inhaled or diffused throughout a room. When bergamot essential oil is experienced as aromatherapy, it may lower blood pressure and improve mental health. These calming properties might be why bergamot is thought to improve sleep.

However, many sleep studies involving bergamot use essential oil mixtures rather than bergamot oil alone, making it difficult to determine the precise effects bergamot essential oil has on sleep. One such study of healthy women found that a mixture of bergamot and sandalwood essential oils improved sleep quality in 64% of study participants. Another study of people in cardiac rehabilitation found that sleep quality significantly increased after exposure to an aromatherapy mixture of bergamot, lavender, and ylang-ylang.

Chamomile

There are two types of chamomile plants: Roman and German. These plant varieties are similar, although they have different combinations of active ingredients and, as a result, potentially different effects. Roman chamomile essential oil is more known for reducing anxiety, while German chamomile is known for relieving pain. If a person experiences anxiety or pain that interferes with sleep, reducing those symptoms could in turn improve sleep.

The effect drinking chamomile tea has on sleep is more commonly studied, but people do engage in chamomile aromatherapy for sleep as well. Roman chamomile, lavender, and neroli is an essential oil blend for sleep that has been scientifically studied. This blend reduced anxiety and improved sleep quality in a study of patients staying in an intensive care unit.

If you would like to reduce anxiety as part of your sleep hygiene routine, chamomile is one of the best essential oils for sleep and anxiety. In one study, inhaling a mixture of chamomile and lavender essential oils reduced anxiety in nurses. There was an even greater reduction when aromatherapy was paired with music. In another study, Roman chamomile aromatherapy reduced anxiety in pregnant women.

Cedarwood

If you enjoy woodsy scents, consider incorporating cedarwood essential oil as you create your ideal bedroom for sleep. Cedarwood oil has a sedative effect due to a chemical compound called cedrol. The sedative effects of cedrol have been studied in both animals and humans. Inhaling an essential oil mixture that contains cedrol has been demonstrated to improve sleep quality in both young, healthy adults and older adults with dementia, likely because it activates the parasympathetic nervous system. Researchers recommend using cedarwood oil for at least 20 nights to see effects. Cedarwood oil, along with other essential oils, may increase total sleep time and reduce early morning awakenings.

Cedarwood oil appears to be versatile, improving sleep in a variety of different types of people. One study focused on women in their 20s, 30s, and 40s living in Japan, Norway, and Thailand. Cedrol had a sedative effect across groups, even though women in different countries had different baseline levels of anxiety and average sleep times.

Clary Sage Oil

Native to southern Europe, clary sage is an herb. Although it isn't the same plant as the popular dried herb sage, it is often used similarly for flavoring foods. Some people may also use clary sage essential oil for its sleep-promoting properties. Studies show that clary sage oil has an antidepressant effect and reduces cortisol levels. Since cortisol impacts circadian rhythms and appears to be tied to alertness, reducing cortisol may promote sleep.

Clary sage may also improve sleep by reducing anxiety. In one study, clary sage oil inhalation appeared to reduce stress in medical patients by lowering their blood pressure and respiratory rate. If anxiety interferes with your ability to sleep and you enjoy the smell of herbs, clary sage oil might be a good option for you.

CHAPTER 4: GUT HEALTH

Another major influence on your immune system is your gut health.

Gut": What Is It?

Everyone has heard about the significance of gut health and gut health, but what exactly is the "gut"? Although some would argue that the whole digestive tract—from ingestion to excretion—is the "gut," the majority of the actual action takes place after the material has been broken down and exited the stomach.

Indeed, the stomach plays a crucial role in the process, but the intestinal system comes to mind when considering the gut, mostly the small intestine, which is responsible for about 90% of nutritional absorption. Many food intolerances also originate in the small intestine. About 70% of people are lactose intolerant, and after consuming a dairy product, they may have diarrhea, nausea, bloating, gas, or stomach discomfort for 30 to 2 hours.

Individuals who are lactose intolerant have trouble digesting milk products because they do not create enough lactase, an enzyme that aids in the breakdown of milk sugars. After ingesting dairy products, undigested lactose remains in the gut and ferments, causing the symptoms that many individuals have.

Therefore, the small intestine is really the major location

of the often reported "stomach ache" or "upset stomach"! The large intestine, also known as the colon, is the primary location for the microbiome—the community of beneficial bacteria—while the small intestine is responsible for nutrition absorption and a host of other processes. In actuality, the intestinal tract contains the whole "gut" that we are all talking about.

Gut Microbiome and Flora

The majority of readers have almost certainly heard the terms "gut flora" and/or "microbiome," but what exactly is the microbiome? And what's meant by gut flora?

All of the bacteria, viruses, fungus, and other tiny creatures that reside in your intestines are together referred to as the microbiome. We refer to those same microorganisms as the gut flora. I know it seems scary, because fungus and bacteria are nasty, right? Not all of them, however. Beneficial microorganisms are essential to bodily processes. Your general health is really primarily dependent on maintaining a healthy gut flora.

The microbiome serves a wide range of purposes. Maintaining a healthy gut flora facilitates digestion by assisting the body in breaking down certain meals that the stomach and small intestine are unable to process. Additionally, gut flora contributes significantly to the immune system by acting as a barrier, stopping the development of dangerous bacteria, and assisting in the synthesis of vitamins B and K.

Studies have even connected the gut-brain axis's health and function to the microbiome. Experts now refer to this microbiota as an "organ," given its primary role in the body's regular operation and the many tasks it performs. Nonetheless, because the microbiome is not innate, it is regarded as an "acquired organ," beginning at birth and changing throughout the course of a person's life.

The total weight of microbiota may reach up to 2 kg (4

lbs). The cecum is a little area of the big intestine that is home to a significant population of these bacteria. The region where the small intestine joins the large intestine, known as the cecum, is pouch-like and located close to the appendix.

Microbes may also be found in the stomach, esophagus, and small intestine, but in much lesser quantities. Healthy intestinal walls will be able to host more of that ideal microbiota than an unhealthy intestinal wall since these microorganisms reside in the mucosal lining of the intestinal wall. In order to increase the amount of good gut flora, several diets and supplements may also be beneficial. These supplements are often probiotics.

Probiotics

For those who have visited health stores, attended natural product exhibits, or read up on health trends, it is evident that prebiotics and probiotics are becoming more and more popular. In 2012 alone, there were about 3 million more persons in the US using probiotic or prebiotic supplements than there were in 2007, a four-fold increase in the usage of these supplements. These figures have only gone up in the last several years. However, you may want to grasp what the distinction is between probiotics and prebiotics before getting too technical.

In actuality, prebiotics and probiotics vary greatly. Dietary components like fiber are referred to as prebiotics because they aid in the development of beneficial bacteria in the stomach. These consist of flaxseeds, apples, oats, garlic, asparagus, and bananas, among other things.

Probiotics, on the other hand, are real, live microorganisms that are said to provide several health advantages, including assistance for the digestive system. Live culture yogurts, fermented meals and drinks, nutritional supplements, and even non-oral items like skin lotions are all marketed as probiotic goods.

Though some people may find the concept of purposefully ingesting germs and microbes unusual or unsettling, the advantages of probiotics have made this notion more popular among the general population. Probiotic bacteria aid in vitamin production, aid in food digestion, and eliminate pathogenic microbes. Furthermore, a large number of the microbes included in probiotic supplements are identical to or comparable to those that our bodies naturally contain in order to carry out these tasks.

Recognize that not all probiotics are created equal while reading about how to choose one. Probiotics include a wide variety of microorganisms that, while belonging to the same family of bacteria, have distinct roles in the body.

For instance, the most prevalent are from the Bifidobacterium and Lactobacillus families. Numerous bacterial species from each of these two groups' respective families are included. If one strain of Lactobacillus bacteria is shown to be protective against a disease, it is not a given that another strain would be as effective. When adding new bacteria to their bodies, those with compromised immune systems or major medical conditions should exercise caution. Apart from probiotics, several dietary supplements may also assist to enhance the intestinal environment and increase the hospitability of beneficial bacteria. In any case, it is essential to speak with a doctor before starting a new nutritional supplement.

Leaky Gut

Increased intestinal permeability, a condition where toxins and germs may seep past the intestinal wall and into the circulation, is essentially what is meant to be understood when one has a leaky gut.

Our food is broken down by the digestive system into usable nutrients, which are then transferred to the bloodstream and distributed throughout the body as required. Furthermore, the digestive system functions as a physical gatekeeper, permitting only useful substances to pass through.

Tight junctions are the name for these gatekeepers. Tiny gaps called tight junctions exist throughout the intestinal wall. They let water and nutrients pass through while blocking the passage of germs and poisons into the circulation. The so-called leaky gut syndrome results from these tight connections becoming loose, which essentially makes the gut wall more permeable to both dangerous bacteria and toxins as well as helpful chemicals. Inadequate circulatory circulation of germs and toxins leads to hyperactive immune response and systemic inflammation. This subsequently causes gastrointestinal bloating, excessive wind, poor digestion, tiredness, underproductivity, and even skin issues—symptoms of a leaky gut.

Many people are still curious about the etiology of leaky gut. Although research on leaky gut syndrome is ongoing, zonulin is assumed to be partially or maybe entirely to blame. The gut may become more permeable if this protein is activated by intestinal bacteria that have seeped out of it. Numerous factors may cause zonulin activity, such as consuming a diet heavy in sugar, using non-steroidal anti-inflammatory medicines (like ibuprofen) for an extended period of time, stress, inflammation, and routinely consuming excessive amounts of alcohol.

We are hearing more about the illness these days as researchers gain better understanding of the gut and its function in immune system and general health. More people are taking responsibility for their own health, reading up on topics, and learning about ailments like leaky guts. We then desire to take action to mend our own intestines after realizing that's maybe what we've had all along. Chronic fatigue syndrome, fibromyalgia, diabetes, Crohn's disease, and a few food allergies have all been linked to leaky gut syndrome. Making every effort to stop and fix a leaky gut may help shield us against long-term illnesses.

Absorption

Absorption is a critical component of gut health that is often disregarded. In the nutrition and supplement sectors, this phrase is often used. However, how many people really get it? The small intestine, which is the primary location of nutrition absorption, is where it all begins. These nutrients need to cross the intestinal lumen, enter the mucosal cells that line the digestive system, and finally enter the circulation in order to be absorbed. Several processes are involved in this, and they vary depending on the kind of nutrient that is flowing through.

First is diffusion. Simply said, this is the movement of molecules from a high concentration location to a lower concentration area. Molecules may effortlessly pass the cell membrane on their own when simple diffusion is occurring.

Osmosis, or the dispersion of water, comes next. Then came enhanced diffusion, in which the nutrient enters the circulation without the requirement for a carrier or transport molecule. The transportation mentioned above are all passive and don't need energy to operate. Additionally, there is active transport, which requires a carrier molecule in addition to energy to be absorbed. In contrast to straightforward passive diffusion, this kind of transport may carry materials from a lower concentration into a greater concentration.

Even though the body naturally absorbs nutrients, having a sick stomach might reduce the amount of nutrients that are really absorbed and used by the body. Certain supplements for gut health may assist to improve this absorption, which will raise the vitamins, proteins, and other vital components in our meals' bioavailability.

Bioavailability

Simply said, bioavailability is the amount of a nutrient that the body can absorb and utilize. The vitamins and minerals we ingest have widely differing levels of bioavailability. Almost all of the sodium we consume is absorbed by the body because some minerals, like sodium, are absorbed at a very high percentage. In contrast, just around 25% of what we consume is usually absorbed when it comes to calcium. Iron has much less, at 5%.

Generally speaking, the body absorbs animal goods more readily than plant ones. This is due to the fact that plants include compounds like fiber, phytates, tannins, and oxalates that bind minerals in the digestive system and limit absorption. Regrettably, the body would benefit from these plant-based diets' increased bioavailability since they include a lot of nutrients.

For instance, turmeric is well known for its antioxidant and anti-inflammatory qualities, yet its bioavailability is often poor. Many firms incorporate compounds that promote absorption to assist the increase of the bioavailability of curcumin, the main chemical in turmeric, so that lesser quantities taken will have a bigger impact. This allows consumers to actually benefit from turmeric's anti-inflammatory properties. Once again, it is critical to consider the impact those gut-enhancing substances have on absorption. Do they swell up to force nutrients through? Or instead, do they collaborate with the stomach to stimulate natural transporters and repair the lining?

A Diet for Gut Health

Our whole health is directly impacted by the condition of our stomach. Immune system strength, mood, and food digestion are all influenced by the integrity of our gut; difficulties with food digestion brought on by a compromised gut may result in inadequate nutrition and even disease.

Our microbiome, a vital collection of billions of bacteria, fungi, and viruses, lives in our stomach. These microbes, also known as "good bacteria," support the proper function of our digestive tract. Furthermore, the microbiome in our stomach affects our skin, immune system, emotional and physical well-being, and risk of contracting illnesses like cancer. Take care of our microbiome, and it will take care of us. Our gut health and microbiota are influenced by the foods we consume, so what should we eat more of and less of to keep our guts healthy?

Pickles, kimchi, sauerkraut, kombucha, yogurt, and kefir are examples of fermented foods and beverages that are excellent for the digestive system. They have probiotic bacteria, which aid in keeping the harmful bacteria out of our digestive tract and helping the healthy bacteria populate it. A particular kind of fiber known as prebiotics is what the microbes in our microbiome love to eat. Prebiotic fibers include inulin, which is found in foods like garlic, onions, and leeks. Good-for-you meals also aid in the absorption of water by the colon, facilitating the easy movement of waste products and food throughout the whole length of the intestines. Fruits, vegetables, legumes, and whole grains fall within this category.

Food that May Impair Gut Health

The adage that fresh veggies and whole grains are healthy while processed red meats, sweets, and saturated fats are unhealthy has a basis that goes beyond heart health and weight control. Sugary, salty, and high-fat diets are terrible for the intestines. As much as possible, steer clear of processed meats, baked goods, desserts, chips, fried meals, and fast food if you want to strengthen the health of your digestive system. Store them as seldom sweets.

And trust your instincts. Many individuals have dietary intolerances to certain proteins, like gluten, or sugars, such lactose, which is present in dairy products. You should stay away from these foods if they make you feel bloated, gassy, or uncomfortable after eating them. You may be intolerant to them. A sick stomach will physically talk to you. As it attempts to process the food you consume, it will gurgle and create sounds that are beyond your control. Along with gas and bloating, you could also feel gastrointestinal aches that go throughout your body. Along with regular weight gain or loss, you could also have diarrhea or constipation.

Digestion is not the only symptom of a sick gut. Because of the gut-brain link, having a bad stomach may cause mood changes, depression, difficulty concentrating, and even skin conditions like eczema. Also, you might have difficulty getting a decent night's sleep, which would leave you feeling drained and agitated all the time. For many people, these symptoms are frequent and daily occurrences, and they are often attributed to other factors like stress or just having a busy life. If this describes you, it may be time to listen to your body and your nutrition. You may regain control over your health and find the correct path to gut health by learning to listen to your body's cues.

What is your gut telling you?

The digestive system's functions include breaking down, or digesting, food, getting rid of impurities, and absorbing energy and other essential elements that our bodies need to operate properly. But it's also significant in other respects.

Gut health's impact on mental health

Additionally, the state of our gut affects our mental and emotional well-being. Poor gut health may also have a negative impact on our mental health. Therefore, maintaining the health of our digestive system is crucial to our general well-being and goes beyond just avoiding digestive illnesses like gas, bloating, and constipation. Fortunately, there are easy things that we can all do to promote gut health.

In addition to the apparent importance of eating and

drinking the correct foods, our digestion is also influenced by the way we exercise our body. It aids in stimulating the stomach and raises digestive activity, to start.

Train to maintain intestinal health

The muscles in our digestive system get more blood flow when we exercise, which massages our food as it passes through the digestive tract, a mechanism called peristalsis, which speeds up and improves the efficiency of their job.

Additionally, studies indicate that exercise modifies the microbiota's equilibrium in the gut. The so-called gut flora actively defends our immune system, inhibits the development of harmful bacteria, and aids in the body's digestion and absorption of nutrients from the food we consume.

Steer clear of intense cardio workouts

During the period of digestion, it is crucial to steer clear of certain high-impact workout kinds, like:

- Dance
- Trampoline
- Kickboxing
- Jogging
- Team sports

Choose walking and other low-impact physical activities instead of these workouts, since they might disturb the digestive system and create pain and stitches.

The Super 3 Peristalsis is a pattern of digestive workouts that helps us digest meals by rubbing food along the digestive canal. It is an involuntary muscular activity in the gut. By aiding this process, this particularly crafted workout program helps improve your digestion.

After a short meal or snack, you may start the program right away; however, if you've had a larger meal, you should wait around half an hour.

To protect your knees while kneeling for the exercises, it is advised that you use an exercise mat or towel.

Workout 1

It's okay to do this workout just after a little lunch or snack. It's crucial that you take your time, so concentrate on moving slowly and deliberately.

Put your hands flat on the floor just under your shoulders as you drop on all fours. Right behind your hips is where your knees should be. Make sure your back is straight.

Stretch your right arm out till it's parallel to your shoulder, very slowly. Elevate your left leg concurrently to align your heel with your hips. Try to draw a straight line that extends from your right arm to your left foot.

After maintaining this posture for a little while, very gently begin to pull in your left knee and right arm to return to the beginning position.

From this position, let your back arch as if a belt is drawing you up, lowering your head and tailbone. Hold this for a brief moment before repeating at least 10 times with the same arm and leg. Repeat after resting on the other side.

After you've finished this program, go directly to the stretches. In addition to massaging the stomach muscles and easing any bloating sensations, they will facilitate the peristalsis process.

Workout 2

You should now be laying on your back on your mat or towel after turning over. All you have to do is fold both of your knees into your chest and give them a little embrace.

Now, while still holding onto the opposite knee, carefully stretch one leg straight out. After that, swap by drawing the straight leg back in.

For the whole exercise, keep your head and shoulders on the floor. Do this ten times.

Workout 3

In order to complete the exercise, return both feet to the floor and gradually extend your legs straight out so that you are resting flat with your arms by your sides.

Keep your arms in touch with the floor as you slowly stretch them out to the side and up beyond your head.

Now extend yourself to your maximum length. Any internal pressure is released as a result. Keep this pose for ten to twenty seconds.

These workouts may even reduce abdominal fat and improve digestion:

Workout 4

Riding a bike is another excellent way to keep the digestive system running smoothly. Not only can cycling promote intestinal health, but it also helps reduce belly fat.

Workout 5

The goal of ab exercise is to strengthen the abdominal muscles and correct the digestive system. This exercise may be tried in a variety of ways, such as the vertical leg crunch, long arm crunch, and reverse crunch. One of the finest workouts for a healthy digestive system is a sit-up or crunch. Your intestines and bowel movement are strengthened by the muscles in your belly and core. Additionally, they aid in avoiding digestive problems including bloating and gas. Better more, this workout may help you get flat abs and decrease belly fat!

Workout 6

You may be surprised to learn that even this basic breathing exercise has an impact on your digestion. An appropriate breathing pattern may assist with issues like bloating and heartburn. All you have to do is practice breathing in and out using your abdominal muscles while sitting up straight. By relaxing, you'll be able to control your stress levels.

Did you know that our gut health may also be significantly impacted by the drugs we take?

The digestive system, including the stomach, small and large intestines, is sometimes referred to as the "gut." About 1,000 different kinds of bacteria, both beneficial and harmful, live in our stomachs. These bacteria help digest food, support immune system function, create essential nutrients, and shield us from infections and poisons. We must maintain the right mix of microorganisms in our guts to be healthy. But that balance may be thrown off by a number of the typical drugs we use.

Diversity of bacteria is essential for a healthy gut. It is a good thing that many of the regular drugs we take, including antibiotics, destroy harmful germs. Regretfully, they also destroy healthy bacteria, or the natural flora of the stomach, which is terrible. To guarantee proper utilization, you should work closely with your doctor and be aware of the prescriptions you're taking.

You should be aware of the following drugs since they may have an impact on gut health:

Antibiotics: Although they are very successful in treating severe bacterial illnesses, abuse and misuse of antibiotics are a cause for worry. When an ailment may heal itself, avoid using antibiotics and never take an antibiotic if your doctor hasn't given it to you.

Nonsteroidal Anti-Inflammatory Drugs (NSAIDs): NSAIDs, such as Aleve, Advil, and Motrin, are the most used pain relievers in America. Sadly, they do more than just dull suffering.

They also throw off the good bacteria's regular equilibrium in your digestive system.

PPIs, or proton pump inhibitors, It is also known that these acid blockers, which are used to treat acid reflux, peptic ulcers, and dyspepsia, reduce the variety of gut flora. This may result in vitamin shortages, bone fractures, and infections such as pneumonia and Clostridium difficile (often referred to as C. difficile or C. diff). Omeprazole, pantoprazole, esomeprazole, lansoprazole, rabeprazole, and dexlansoprazole are some examples of generic PPI names.

Antacids: In general, antacids (not only PPIs) neutralize stomach acid, the body's first line of defense against hazardous bacteria that we encounter on a daily basis. If we use antacids often, we increase our risk of infections and stomach bugs. Researchers discovered unusually significant concentrations of bacteria, which are typically exclusively located in the mouth cavity, in the colons of patients on gastric acid medications. When germs from the mouth cavity attempt to enter the stomach, where they shouldn't be, stomach acid often destroys them. However, when you take these stomach acid inhibitors, this is not the case. This is significant because oral bacteria in the colon is linked to an increased risk of developing certain types of colon cancer.

Antidepressants: Selective serotonin reuptake inhibitors (SSRIs) are among the most widely used kinds of antidepressants. An estimated 90% of serotonin is produced in the stomach, according to scientists. Osteoporosis, cardiovascular disease, and irritable bowel syndrome have all been related to serotonin imbalances.

Sleeping pills: These medications are fat-soluble, much as antidepressants. They have the ability to pierce the intestinal membrane and disrupt the digestive system's normal equilibrium.

Laxatives: The equilibrium of gut flora may also be

impacted by laxatives. They need to be used sparingly and only under a doctor's or other health care provider's supervision.

Statins: The most often prescribed drugs globally are statins, or cholesterol-lowering drugs. The balance of intestinal flora may be adversely affected by statins, according to recent studies. There is a need for further research.

If you have any concerns about how your medications may be affecting your gut health, always talk to your physician. Never abruptly cease using a prescription drug that you have been given. The right balance between the possible hazards and the benefits of a prescription drug can only be determined by your physician.

Consider your stomach as a garden. To help grow beneficial bacteria, fill it with wholesome, high-fiber foods like fruit, vegetables, whole grains, and legumes. Avoid processed meat, sugar, and fatty foods, which encourage the growth of bad bacteria. A strong stomach can only be maintained by regular Exercise and drinking plenty of water. Seven to ten eight-ounce glasses of water each day make for a good general guideline, but individual needs vary. We can all take a lot of action to promote our overall health by preserving the right variety of bacteria in the gut microbiome.

Fortunately, not all medications have a negative impact on gut health. One startling findings was proof that two widely prescribed medications, blood pressure medication (also known as beta-blockers) and diuretic tablets (also known as loop diuretics) together, are linked to higher concentrations of the bacterium Roseburia, which is known to promote health.

This particular kind of bacteria has the ability to break down plant-based dietary fiber and produce butyric acid, which has many health advantages including reducing inflammation and controlling the epigenome. That is our DNA's dynamic portion.

Individuals with cardiovascular disease who were also taking statins, a popular family of medications that decrease blood levels of dangerous LDL cholesterol, were also more likely to have a better mix of different gut flora. The discovery that the combination of statins and cardiac magnesium was linked to decreased blood levels of dangerous lipids was very intriguing.

The amount of bacteria in the stomach may be directly altered by probiotics and prebiotics. Your digestive tract may be replenished with the nutrition it needs to generate digestive enzymes efficiently with the help of vitamins and minerals.

The lengthy layer of cells that line the digestive canal that may become inflamed and damaged over time due to disruptions in the gut microbiota can also be healed by some nutrients. This may result in intestinal permeability, sometimes referred to as "leaky gut," a condition where the cells lining the stomach allow poisons and allows other chemicals to enter the bloodstream and tax the immune system.

To gradually promote balance in the gut microbiome, probiotics and prebiotics in particular work best when taken consistently, possibly for several weeks.

Supplements for Intestinal Health

Probiotics are live, healthy yeasts and bacteria that you may ingest via supplements or fermented meals. The amount of bacteria currently living in the gut may be increased by supplementing with probiotics.

By competitive exclusion, or edging out, some strains or species of probiotics may prevent the proliferation of harmful microbes. This improves the environment and allows the healthy bacteria that are already there to proliferate.

Probiotics have the ability to boost immunity as well. Two of the most prevalent kinds of bacteria in the stomach, lactobacilli and bifidobacteria, help lessen leaky gut by preserving the integrity of the gut lining that harmful bacteria erode.

Prebiotics

Prebiotics are indigestible fibers found in food that support healthy gut flora. Gut bacteria break down prebiotic fiber during fermentation to create beneficial metabolites including short-chain fatty acids that are good for your gut. These substances are then used by the lining of your stomach to grow and remain strong. These substances may also be distributed throughout the remainder of your body, where they can help regulate cholesterol and your cardiovascular system, among other things.

Fiber

Fiber provides plants with structure, which explains why carrots and apples have such a delightful crunch. Fiber is able to enter the colon and help facilitate regular, pleasant bowel movements because it is resistant to being broken down by the digestive enzymes. Along the journey, fiber may support the growth of gut microorganisms, absorb substances that the stool will excrete, and keep the stool's water content stable enough to facilitate passage.

By decreasing the pace at which nutrients enter the circulation, soluble fiber may support metabolic health by fostering feelings of fullness, blood sugar control, and even weight management. To support the maintenance of the body's hormonal balance, fiber may even aid in the proper excretion of hormone metabolites, such as those associated with estrogen.

Just 5% of Americans consume the required amounts of fiber, meaning that most do not. An adult should consume 28–36 grams of fiber on average. Eating more plant foods, which are naturally high in fiber in their least processed form can help you boost your intake of fiber. Another quick and easy strategy to increase your consumption of fiber is to take fiber supplements.

Collagen

Collagen is not just a vitamin for healthy hair, skin, and nails—it may also promote intestinal health.

The stomach lining may become stronger with collagen. One of the primary building blocks of connective tissues, such as blood vessels, skin, tendons, bones, and the lining of the digestive system, is this protein. Glycine is an amino acid necessary for the reconstruction of the tissue lining along the digestive track, is abundant in collagen. Through its functions as an immune system stimulant and antioxidant, glycine may also function as a neurotransmitter in the central nervous system, which may help the gut by way of the gut-brain axis.

By increasing the number of bacteria that stimulate the creation of short chain fatty acids, which are substances that support the health of gut cells, collagen may also function similarly to prebiotic fibers.

In research of healthy women, the majority of the participants reported less bloating and other digestive issues after taking 10g dosages of collagen twice day for eight weeks.

Zinc

Based on preliminary study, zinc may have advantages since it helps to maintain a healthy immune system and robust intestinal lining. This mineral may enhance the immune system's ability to fight off harmful intestinal bacteria and even aid in the process of apoptosis, which is the recycling of cells.

The synthesis of digestive enzymes also depends on sufficient zinc levels. According to research on animals, consuming insufficient amounts of zinc via diet might affect the production of pancreatic enzymes.

For most individuals, the Recommended Dietary Allowance (RDA) for zinc is 8–11 mg.

Licorice Root

Because of its flavonoid concentration, licorice root may help soothe the digestive tract and lessen occasional discomfort and inflammation.

As licorice root itself has blood pressure-raising characteristics, it would be advisable to consume it as DGL (deglycyrrhizinated licorice).

When is the optimum time to take supplements for gut health?

For the majority of the supplements mentioned above to have cumulative effects, regular use is recommended.

For occasional usage in cases of dyspepsia, licorice root may be used.

Since zinc may sometimes upset the stomach when taken on an empty stomach, it is best to take zinc with meals. However, because iron and calcium supplements may interfere with the absorption of zinc, take zinc on its own.

Potential Adverse Affects

The above-discussed gut health supplements have very little risk. However, licorice root may cause an increase in blood pressure; however, this impact is lessened when taken as DGL, or deglycyrrhizinated form.

Some individuals may experience bloating and changes in stool consistency after taking probiotics and prebiotics. Altering the probiotic strains or lowering the dosage are two options you may explore. Since various prebiotics feed different bacteria in the stomach, switching to a different kind of prebiotic could be beneficial. It would be preferable to lower the dosage and then increase it gradually over a few weeks to allow your gut bacteria time to stabilize.

Who shouldn't use vitamins for gut health?

For the most part, probiotics, prebiotics, fiber, and collagen are safe. The ideal people for zinc are those who have a verified shortage, may not obtain enough from their diet, or have gastrointestinal conditions that make absorption difficult.

Because there is insufficient evidence to support its safe and effective usage, licorice is not recommended for use by pregnant or nursing mothers.

How long do vitamins for gut health take to start working?

Certain vitamins could provide immediate assistance. It might take a little longer with other vitamins before you start to see any changes.

Probiotics and prebiotics work best when taken regularly, ideally for a few weeks at least, to gradually restore equilibrium to the gut microbiota. Keep an eye on how these supplements are making you feel and note any changes to your bowel and digestive processes.

The average period to restore gut health when adhering to a customized strategy might be around three months. It could be beneficial to consult with a healthcare provider who specializes in gut health if you have struggled to manage recurrent gastrointestinal issues.

Of course, everybody experiences stress, but when stress becomes overwhelming or too persistent then it can have a wide range of negative consequences, including a negative impact on gut health.

Between 70 and 80 percent of all diseases and ailments are stress-related, and lifestyle diseases are the primary cause of mortality. However, we do not need statistics to tell us that when we neglect ourselves, we feel anxious, fatigued, and creatively drained. Below is a list of one hundred strategies to alleviate tension.

Environmental Techniques

The first area to investigate for stress-reduction strategies is your immediate environment.

What are you able to see, sense, hear, feel, and taste? What causes you to lower your shoulders and exclaim "Ahhhh"? Consider methods to add elegance to your surroundings. Here are a few items to help you get started:

1. Have fun just being

2. Light a scented candle

3. Aromatherapy

4. Baking

5. Adjust lighting

6. Plant flowers

7. Buy yourself a bouquet.

8. Create a collection of things you love

9. Put up a bird feeder and observe the birds

10. Read in the sunshine

11. Sip a heated or cold drink

12. Snuggle up with a book under a comforter.

Cognitive Techniques

The second domain to target when reducing stress is how you process and interpret information. Your emotional response is determined by your mental interpretations, so ruminating on problems, imagining the worst-case scenario, and berating yourself for errors will all increase your tension levels. Alternately, allowing yourself to make blunders and moving on, considering the best-case scenario, and interpreting errors as learning opportunities will reduce stress.

Here are some cognitive stress-reduction strategies:

13. Reframe the issue

14. Be positive

15. Meditate on positive words

17. Practice positive affirmations

18. Maintain reasonable expectations

19. Visualize the desired outcome.

20. Display affirmations on a mirror

21. Solve a riddle or game

Innovative Techniques

Creativity is an excellent method for transforming tension into loveliness. Utilize the arts to both unwind and process your difficulties. Process is more essential than product. These are some inventive techniques for relieving stress:

22. Write in a journal

23. Write a letter

24. Paint

25. Draw

26. Spend an afternoon photographing

27.. Create pottery/work with clay

28. Knit/Crochet/Needlework

29. Pet a pet

30. Listen to/compose relaxing music

31. Play an instrument

32. Attend a concert

33. Begin a new passion

34. Garden

Physical Techniques

Frequent physical manifestations of stress include tense muscles, apprehensive movement, and rigidity. Stretching, aerobic exercise, and rhythmic motion can be utilized to relieve tension. Care for your body by making nutritious dietary choices. Try the following to physically reduce stress:

35. Dance

36. Ride a Bike

37. Run

38. Walk/hike in nature

39. Walk the dog

40. Train for a walking/marathon fundraiser

41. Swim.

42. Snorkel.

43. Get a massage.

44. Give yourself a foot massage

45. Soak your feet in warm water

46. Enjoy a steamy bubble bath

47. Take a yoga class

48. Practice t'ai chi

49. Do progressive muscular relaxation

50. Frequently practice deep breathing

51. Watch an exercise video

52. Eat a healthy diet

53. Drink water

Humorous Techniques

55. See a comedy film.

56. View a humorous sitcom

57. Read a comic book.

58. Laugh out loud

59. Tell a friend a joke

60. Laugh with a friend

Spiritual Techniques

We are holistic creatures, and our spiritual nature can also help alleviate tension. Try the following spiritual preventive measures for stress:

61. Pray

62. Meditate

63. Practice gratitude

64. Take part in a religious service

65. Sing joyful songs/hymns

66. Seek opportunities to serve others

Management Techniques

Due to procrastination, disorganization, and lack of attention to the smallest of details, some tension is created or exacerbated. By organizing your time, money, plans, and debris, you can alter your mood in as little as 15 minutes. Some management strategies include:

67. Time management

68. task prioritization

69. Delegate

70. Create and adhere to a budget

71. Solve one problem

72. Clean a room

73. Organize a cabinet or closet

74. Set objectives

75. Create a life list

76. Visualize achievement

Relationship Techniques

As long as we interact with others, relational tension will exist. This is even more vital in relationships that are meaningful to us. However, just as relationships can cause tension, they can also alleviate it. Try these relationship techniques to reduce stress:

77. Cook a special meal for a loved one

78. Be politely assertive

79. Vent to a friend.

80. Meet someone for lunch/coffee.

81. Call a friend

82. Get a manicure

83. Get a haircut

84. Email a friend

85. Join a social-support group

86. Join a fitness class or group

87. Forgive an offense

88. Volunteer

89. Do something just for fun

Outdoor Techniques

Being outdoors can alter our disposition by literally giving us a new perspective. Regardless of the weather or climate, you can implement outdoor stress relief strategies for a fast or leisurely activity. The following outdoor strategies may prove useful:

90. Sit on a park bench and use the senses

91. Stroll through a zoo or aquarium

92. Star gaze

93. Spend some time boating or sailing

94. Take a scenic drive

95. Build a sandcastle

96. Build a snowman

97. Hear the crackling of a campfire

98. Have a picnic near water

99. Eat dinner out

100. Window shop

In conclusion

Now you have a list of 100 ways to reduce tension, but they will be ineffective if they remain on paper. Choose at least one and use it immediately. Create a plan (management strategy) to implement one stress management technique per day for the next week. Combining a physical and external strategy, take a vigorous 10-minute walk outside.

Throughout this book, food has been a common topic, but now we will take a more in-depth look at which foods promote healthy digestion and which foods might harm it.

Gut health is a complex topic, and conflicting recommendations online can make it challenging to understand which foods are best for supporting a balance of beneficial gut bacteria.

Below you'll find a gut health grocery list with tips for how you can start shopping for foods that support healthy digestion.

For individualized advice and meal planning help to improve your gut health, consider booking a call with a registered dietitian.

Gut Health Grocery List Basics

When writing a grocery list for digestive health, the first step is understanding how different foods and eating patterns can impact the gut microbiome (all of the bacteria in your digestive system).

Your digestive tract contains trillions of bacteria, and many factors, including food choices, can influence the types of bacteria present. When planning your grocery list for gut health, you'll want to include foods from the following categories for a nutritionally complete diet:

- Complex carbohydrates for energy and fiber.
- Protein for satiety.
- Fruits and vegetables for vitamins, minerals, antioxidants, and fiber.
- Healthy fats for satiety and vitamin absorption.
- Pantry staples and frozen goods for convenience.

What is Dysbiosis?

Dysbiosis occurs when there is a disproportionate level of harmful bacteria in your gut. It can result in gastrointestinal symptoms like bloating, upset stomach, and gas. It may also cause inflammation and impact immune function, which has been linked to an increased risk of chronic conditions like diabetes, obesity, and cancer.

Research shows that people who follow a Mediterranean diet have greater levels of health-promoting gut bacteria and a lower risk of chronic diseases. This diet consists of minimally processed foods, fruits, vegetables, legumes, healthy fats, whole grains, and limited amounts of animal products.

In addition, food sources of prebiotics and probiotics benefit gut health. Prebiotics, like onions, asparagus, and oats, act as food sources for your healthy gut bacteria to grow.

Probiotics, on the other hand, are foods or supplements that contain live active cultures (good bacteria) and are typically found in cultured or fermented foods, like yogurt, kefir, sauerkraut, and kimchi.

Foods to Include for Gut Health

When considering the foods to include or exclude from your diet, it's important to understand that one size does not fit all. If you've been diagnosed with a specific gastrointestinal disorder, there may be a different set of dietary guidelines to help your symptoms.

For example, people with irritable bowel syndrome (IBS) may need to limit certain types of fiber, while those with celiac disease must avoid gluten. If you have chronic digestive symptoms, talk to your doctor to determine the underlying cause before making major dietary changes.

A doctor or registered dietitian can help guide your food choices to support gut health based on your medical history, symptoms, and food intolerances or allergies.

Protein

Research shows that a high intake of animal proteins, especially red meat and certain kinds of dairy, can increase harmful gut bacteria. Plant-based proteins have a protective effect and help support the growth of health-promoting bacteria in the digestive tract. Some health proteins include:

- Beans, like pinto beans, garbanzo beans, and black beans.
- Lentils, including red lentils, brown lentils, and green lentils.
- Peas, such as split peas and yellow peas.
- Soy protein, such as tofu, edamame, and tempeh.
- Poultry, like chicken and turkey.
- Fish, including salmon and tuna.
- Eggs.
- Cultured dairy, like yogurt, kefir, and probiotic cottage cheese.

Carbohydrates

Some carbohydrates contain fermentable dietary fiber, meaning bacteria can digest it in the large intestine, supporting a healthy gut microbiome. This type of fiber is primarily found in whole-grain foods.

On the other hand, refined carbohydrates and sugar can negatively impact gut health. Though gluten is commonly excluded in eating plans for gut health, research actually shows a gluten-free diet may decrease the number of healthy gut bacteria. However, it may be important for those with certain diagnoses, such as Celiac disease, to avoid gluten. Here are some healthy carbohydrates you might want to consider adding to your diet:

- Barley.
- Farro.
- Amaranth.

Wheat, such as wheat berries, whole wheat pasta, and

whole wheat bread.

- Rye.
- Brown rice.
- Oats.
- Quinoa.
- Corn.
- Potatoes.

Healthy Fats

There is evidence that a high-fat diet consisting of primarily saturated fats (common in Western diets) can negatively impact the balance of gut bacteria and increase inflammation. Therefore, focusing on monounsaturated fats and omega-3 polyunsaturated fats is best for the gut microbiome. Here are some examples of health fats:

- Extra virgin olive oil.
- Avocados and avocado oil.
- Nuts and nut butters, like peanuts, walnuts, and almonds.
- Seeds, like chia seeds, flax seeds, hemp seeds, and sunflower seeds.
- Fatty fish, like salmon, trout, and tuna.

Fruits

Fruits are rich in polyphenols, which are beneficial plant compounds naturally found in certain foods. Research has linked a higher polyphenol intake with an increase in the number of healthy gut bacteria.

Fruits also contain antioxidants, which have anti-inflammatory properties that support gut health. All fruits are a good source of fiber, and many have prebiotic fiber, which helps your good bacteria grow. These include:

Berries, like blueberries, strawberries, and blackberries.

- Mango.
- Citrus, like oranges, grapefruit, and clementines.
- Grapes.
- Cherries.
- Papaya.
- Pineapple.
- Apricots.
- Peaches.
- Apples.
- Kiwis.

Vegetables

Like fruits, vegetables are excellent sources of gut-friendly antioxidants. Vegetables contain prebiotic fiber, which is important food for healthy gut bacteria. Pickled vegetables are a great source of probiotics, which help introduce health-promoting bacteria to your digestive tract. Here are some examples of some vegetables that support digestive health:

- Bell pepper.
- Beets.
- Cauliflower.
- Broccoli.
- Leafy greens, like spinach, romaine, and kale.
- Winter squash, including butternut squash, pumpkin, and acorn squash.
- Carrots.
- Artichoke.
- Onion.
- Asparagus.
- Brussels sprouts.
- Mushrooms.

- Pickled vegetables, including kimchi, sauerkraut, and probiotic pickles.

Pantry Staples

Consider always keeping your kitchen stocked with the following pantry staples so that you always have the basic ingredients to create a homemade meal. Then, you can supplement this list with fresh foods from the above lists, like fruits, vegetables, avocados, cultured dairy, and lean proteins.

- Dried beans and lentils.
- Frozen, unflavored fruits and vegetables.
- Olive oil.
- Grains, like farro, quinoa, and barley.
- Oats.
- Whole wheat or bean-based pasta.
- Potatoes.
- Nuts, seeds, and nut butters.
- Onions.
- Garlic.
- Pickled vegetables.
- Chicken, beef, or vegetable broth.
- Dried herbs and spices.
- Brown or wild rice.

Foods to Avoid

Conflicting information exists online, recommending people avoid foods like soy, gluten, and legumes for gut health. However, the evidence does not support eliminating these foods from a healthy person's diet to improve digestive function.

Of course, some people may have individual intolerances or conditions requiring avoidance of some of these foods.

Though dairy is often on lists of foods to avoid for gut dysfunction, the data is mixed. While a few small studies show milk may increase certain types of harmful bacteria, other evidence has found the type of fat present in dairy may benefit gut health. In addition, cultured dairy products are an important source of probiotics for many people.

Research has linked certain foods to the growth of harmful bacteria, including:

- Refined grains, like white rice and products made with white flour.
- Added sugars.
- Red meat.
- Processed meats, such as bacon, sausage, and pepperoni.
- Saturated fats, found in foods like butter and fried foods.
- Ultra-processed foods, like chips, soda, and fast food.
- Artificial sweeteners.
- Alcohol.

If you've ever "gone with your gut" to make a decision or felt "butterflies in your stomach" when anxious, it's likely that you're receiving signals from an unexpected source: your second brain. This "brain in your gut" is revolutionizing the medical community's understanding of the connections between digestion, temperament, health, and even the way you think.

This tiny brain is referred to by scientists as the enteric nervous system (ENS). And it is not so small. From the esophagus to the rectum, the ENS consists of two layers of more than 100 million nerve cells lining the gastrointestinal tract.

What Does the Brain of Your Gut Control?

Unlike the large brain in your head, the ENS is incapable of balancing your checkbook or writing a love letter. Its primary function is to regulate digestion, from swallowing to the release of enzymes that break down food to the regulation of blood flow that aids in nutrient absorption and elimination. The enteric nervous system does not appear to be capable of thought as we understand it, but it communicates with our large brain to profound effect.

People contending with irritable bowel syndrome (IBS) and functional bowel problems such as constipation, diarrhea, bloating, pain, and gastrointestinal distress may experience significant emotional alterations when have these problems caused, at least in part, by the ENS. For decades, scientists and physicians believed that anxiety and depression contributed to these conditions. However, recent research indicates that it may also be the other way around. Researchers are discovering evidence that gastrointestinal irritation may transmit signals to the central nervous system (CNS) that induce mood changes.

These new findings may explain why a higher-than-normal percentage of people with IBS and functional bowel problems develop depression and anxiety. Approximately 30 to 40 percent of the population experiences functional gastrointestinal problems at some point.

New Gut Understanding Equals New Treatment Opportunities

This new understanding of the relationship between the ENS and CNS helps to explain the efficacy of IBS and bowel-disorder treatments such as antidepressants and mind-body therapies such as cognitive behavioral therapy (CBT) and medical hypnotherapy. Our two brains 'talk' to each other, so therapies that help one brain may also help the other. In a sense, gastroenterologists (doctors who specialize in digestive disorders) are similar to therapists who seek methods to calm the second brain.

Gastroenterologists may prescribe certain antidepressants for irritable bowel syndrome (IBS) — not because they believe the problem is all in a patient's mind, but because these medications may alleviate symptoms by acting on nerve cells in the stomach. Psychological interventions such as CBT may also help to enhance communications between the large brain and the gut brain.

Could Probiotics Boost Your Mood?

We now understand that a balanced diet is essential for physical health. Researchers are investigating whether probiotics, which are safe, ingestible bacteria, can enhance gastrointestinal health and wellbeing, thus enhancing mental health.

Still More to Understand About Mind-Gut Connection

Research indicates that digestive system activity may also influence cognition (thinking abilities and memory). This is an area that requires more research.

Another area of interest is determining how signals from the digestive system impact the metabolism, thereby increasing or decreasing the risk for type 2 diabetes. This involves interactions between nerve signals, gut hormones, and microbiota—the bacteria that live in the digestive system.

The future of mental health could very well lie in the gut.

CHAPTER 5: WEIGHT

Being overweight or simply being unhealthy, such as having high cholesterol can negatively impact your immune system. In this chapter, we will talk about diets and weight control.

The Mediterranean diet consists almost entirely of foods that come from plants.

Oldways is an organization that, along with the Harvard T.H. Chan School of Public Health and the World Health Organization, created the Mediterranean diet pyramid 25 years ago. At the top of the pyramid are the core foods, which include whole grains, fruits, vegetables, beans, herbs, spices, nuts, and olive oil. The organizations suggest consuming fish and seafood on a twice-weekly basis in addition to moderate amounts of dairy products, eggs, and poultry. Only on occasion would consumers indulge in red meat and sweets.

What are the Advantages and Detriments of Following a Mediterranean Diet?

If you're on the fence about adopting a diet more typical of the Mediterranean, you should think about the studies that support the idea. According to the findings of a study and a meta-analysis, an individual's likelihood of dying from any cause is reduced by five percent for every point that is added to their Mediterranean diet score on a scale that ranges from one to nine.

A study that involved over 26,000 women found that those who followed the Mediterranean diet the most closely had up to a 28 percent lower risk of developing heart disease. The researchers believe that the diet's ability to reduce inflammation may be a key factor in its protective effect. In addition, the antioxidant food component known as hydroxytyrosol, which may be found in foods that are staples of the diet (fruits, nuts, and extra-virgin olive oil), has been demonstrated to repair heart-harming free radical damage, according to the authors of the study.

Even if you don't place a high priority on living a long life and taking care of your heart, there is no ignoring the possibility that you could be interested in the Mediterranean diet due to the possible weight loss it offers. This kind of eating may help you maintain your weight without making you feel deprived, despite the fact that this is not the primary purpose of the strategy.

A study that was conducted by researchers from Harvard University and Emory University followed a group of overweight or obese adults on the Mediterranean diet and a control group eating a standard American diet supplemented with fish oil, walnuts, and grape juice — foods that supply key nutrients in the Mediterranean diet — for a period of eight weeks. A standard American diet is rich in foods that are high in saturated fat, added sugar, and salt. The Mediterranean diet is rich in foods that are low in these three categories. In comparison to the control group, those who followed the Mediterranean diet experienced greater weight loss, a reduction in the blood levels of inflammatory markers, and a decrease in both their total cholesterol and LDL ("bad") cholesterol levels. A pleasant surprise was that this wasn't supposed to be a study on weight loss in the first place (that was just an added benefit), so researchers made sure both groups consumed the same amount of calories.

When it comes to controlling chronic conditions such as type 2 diabetes, dietitians frequently suggest adopting a dietary pattern that is inspired by the Mediterranean. The American

Heart Association notes that this diet is considered heart-healthy despite the fact that it contains more fat than is typically recommended (though it is still low in unhealthy saturated fat).

The main takeaway is that this is one of the healthiest ways you can eat, but as with anything else, you should always talk to your doctor before changing your diet or using a diet as part of your treatment plan for a disease.

5 Suggestions to Help You Get Started on Your Own Mediterranean Diet Plan

Because this is a method of eating rather than a strict set of rules, the good news is that you are free to modify it in any way you see fit to accommodate your preferences for food and drink. There is no way to adhere to this to the letter without risking falling off the bandwagon and experiencing feelings of inadequacy. Even within the Mediterranean diet there are what we call 'special occasion days,' where you may eat more or eat foods that perhaps are not very healthy, but that is actually part of the lifestyle. A healthy connection with food is encouraged by the Mediterranean diet, which recognizes that food is meant to be enjoyed. The term "cheating" refers to a component of the Mediterranean diet. You merely go about your business the following day as if nothing had happened.

Nevertheless, in order to get you started, here are five key pieces of advice:

Eat a diet high in beans. Not only are they a pantry staple that you probably aren't eating enough of anyway, but they are also budget-friendly and offer a plethora of nutritional benefits, such as being high in fiber and protein, low in fat, and a source of B vitamins, iron, and antioxidants. Lentils, dried peas, beans, and chickpeas (such those used to make hummus) are examples of these foods.

Avoid drinking too much alcohol. One of the most popular misconceptions about folks who follow the Mediterranean diet is that they consume a great deal of red wine. The consumption of wine as part of the Mediterranean diet is done so in moderation, and it is always consumed with food. It was common practice to drink only a little amount of wine with meals, typically between three and four ounces.

Cook the meat as a side dish. In the past, people only ate meat on special occasions, such as a Sunday meal, and even then they only ate a limited amount of it on those occasions. You should make an effort to eat more vegetarian main courses throughout the day, such as those that are based on beans, tofu, or seitan. When you do eat meat, choose lean cuts like chicken without the skin and limit your consumption of red meat to once a week or twice a month at most.

Consume fewer sugary foods. Treat sweets like you would meat and save them for rare occasions but on a daily basis, there isn't much sugar eaten. This does not mean that sugar is forbidden; for instance, you can put some in your coffee if you want to.

Olive oil is great to cook with. The best oil for cooking is extra-virgin olive oil, so always use that. Because olive oil is high in heart-healthy monounsaturated and polyunsaturated fats, you may feel good about keeping a bottle of it on hand in the kitchen even though using too much of it might cause weight gain (it is, after all, a fat, so the calories can mount up quickly).

A Comprehensive Food List for the Mediterranean Diet

When attempting to make your diet more Mediterranean, the following foods should be included and others should be avoided:

Protein

Liberally

- Beans
- Lentils

- Chickpeas
- Tofu
- Tempeh
- Seitan

Occasionally

- Chicken
- Fish
- Seafood
- Eggs

Rarely or Never

- Red meat (beef and pork)
- Cured meats (bacon, sausage, and salami)
- Processed meat products (chicken nuggets)

Oil and Fat

Liberally

- Extra-virgin olive oil
- Avocadoes and avocado oil
- Olives

Occasionally

- Canola oil

Rarely or Never

- Trans fats
- Margarine
- Butter

Fruits and Veggies

Liberally

- Nonstarchy veggies, (zucchini, eggplant, bell

peppers, artichokes, and dark greens)
- Starchy veggies (sweet potatoes, potatoes, and root vegetables)
- All fruits (peaches, cherries, apricots, strawberries, raspberries, blueberries, and blackberries)

Occasionally

- There are no off-limits fruits or vegetables.

Rarely or Never

- No fruits or veggies are off-limits.

Nuts and Seeds

Liberally

- While they can be part of every day, eat them in moderation.

Occasionally

- Almonds
- Pistachios
- Hazelnuts
- Walnuts
- Cashews (and all other unsweetened nuts)

Rarely or Never

- Sweetened trail mixes
- Sweetened nut butters
- Sugar-coated nuts

Grains

Liberally

- Whole-grain bread (look for whole-wheat flour as the first ingredient)
- Whole grains (farro, bulgur wheat, barley, and quinoa)

- Oatmeal (steel-cut or old-fashioned)

Occasionally

- Pasta (choose whole-wheat pasta whenever possible)
- Couscous
- Whole-grain crackers
- Polenta
- All-bran cereals

Rarely or Never

- Frozen waffles and pancakes
- Sugar-sweetened cereals
- Crackers and other snack foods

Dairy

Occasionally

- Plain Greek yogurt
- Plain ricotta and cottage cheese
- Milk
- Brie, feta, or goat cheese (plus other cheeses that you enjoy)

Rarely or Never

- Ice cream
- Sweetened yogurt
- Processed cheese (like American)

Sweeteners

Occasionally

- Honey
- A small amount of added sugar (in coffee or tea, for example)

Rarely or Never

- White sugar

Condiments and Sauces

Liberally

- Tomato sauce (no sugar added)
- Pesto
- Balsamic vinegar

Occasionally

- Aioli
- Tahini
- Tzatziki

Rarely or Never

- Barbecue sauce
- Ketchup
- Teriyaki sauce

Drinks

Liberally

- Water
- Coffee
- Tea

Occasionally

- Red wine or other alcohol

Rarely or Never

- Soda
- Fruit juice
- Bottled sweetened coffee

Herbs and Spices

Liberally

- All dried herbs and spices
- All fresh herbs
- Garlic

Occasionally

- Salting food to taste

Your Guide to Following the Mediterranean Diet for the Next 14 Days

When it comes to arranging your menu, here are some suggestions for where to get started. Please take into consideration portion quantities aren't provided. Calorie counting is not required while following this particular diet plan. Your body has unique requirements, and those of another individual won't match up with them.

Day 1

Breakfast Coffee or tea with a bowl of oatmeal topped with berries

Snack Handful of almonds or walnuts

Lunch Half of a turkey sandwich made with whole-grain bread and a cup of lentil soup

Snack Sliced carrots, bell peppers, and cucumbers dipped in hummus

Dinner Veggie and white bean stew

Day 2

Breakfast Coffee or tea with plain Greek yogurt topped with a drizzle of honey and walnuts

Snack Roasted chickpeas

Lunch Leftover veggie and bean stew from yesterday's dinner

Snack A peach (or apple, depending on the season)

Dinner Roasted chicken served with pita bread, tzatziki (a yogurt-based sauce), and a side salad

Day 3

Breakfast Smoothie made with the milk of your choice, fruit, and nut butter

Snack ¼ avocado mashed with lemon juice and salt on top of whole-grain crackers

Lunch Three-bean soup topped with a dollop of pesto and served with a whole-grain roll

Snack Package of olives and fresh veggies

Dinner Salmon with farro and roasted zucchini and eggplant

Day 4

Breakfast Coffee or tea and toasted whole-grain bread, sliced cheese, and strawberries

Snack Pistachios

Lunch Lentil-based salad with feta, roasted red peppers, sun-dried tomatoes, and olives

Snack Greek yogurt with fresh fruit

Dinner Grilled shrimp served with sautéed kale and polenta

Day 5

Breakfast Coffee or tea and a breakfast bowl of leftover farro (from dinner on day 3) topped with a poached egg and a few slices of avocado

Snack Dried apricots and walnuts

Lunch Quinoa, bean, and veggie salad served with a slice of whole-grain bread

Snack Whole-grain crackers and black bean dip

Dinner Marinated, grilled chicken skewers served with bulgur wheat and a cucumber and red onion salad

Day 6

Breakfast Coffee or tea and smoked salmon, capers, and tomato slices

Snack In-season fruit (such as a peach or two apricots in summer, or a pear in winter)

Lunch Mediterranean bean salad and whole-grain crackers

Snack Piece of cheese and olives

Dinner Moroccan lamb stew with couscous

Day 7

Breakfast Coffee or tea and Greek yogurt with sunflower seeds and raspberries

Snack Sliced orange and pistachios

Lunch A piece of whole-grain bread with sliced tomatoes, cheese, and olives

Snack Packaged, flavored lupini beans

Dinner Red lentil and vegetable stew

Day 8

Breakfast Coffee or tea and two eggs with sautéed greens (spinach or kale), plus an orange

Snack Roasted chickpeas

Lunch Leftover lamb stew from dinner on

Day 9

Snack Mixed nuts with a piece of dark chocolate

Dinner Baked white fish, roasted potatoes, and zucchini

Day 10

Breakfast Smoothie made with the milk of your choice, frozen cherries, banana, and cocoa powder

Snack Mini peppers stuffed with hummus

Lunch Tuna salad made with olive oil, dried herbs, olives, and sun-dried tomatoes served on a bed of spinach with mixed veggies and whole-grain crackers

Snack Piece of cheese with a piece of fruit

Dinner Hearty Tuscan white bean soup with whole-grain bread

Day 11

Breakfast Coffee or tea and a bowl of oatmeal topped with raisins and crushed walnuts, plus a drizzle of honey, if desired

Snack Greek yogurt and a piece of fruit

Lunch Leftover Tuscan white bean soup from dinner on day 9

Snack Hummus with sliced raw veggies like red peppers, celery, and cucumber

Dinner Garlic lemon chicken thighs served with asparagus and Israeli couscous

Day 12

Breakfast Coffee or tea and a slice of veggie frittata with avocado

Snack Apple with nut butter

Lunch Prepared dolmas (look for these stuffed grape leaves in the prepared food section at some grocers) with hummus and pita

Snack Greek yogurt dip with sliced veggies

Dinner Seafood stew (shrimp and white fish in a tomato

base)

Day 13

Breakfast Coffee or tea and a small bowl of ricotta topped with fruit (berries, peaches, or fresh apricots) and a drizzle of honey

Snack Handful of lightly salted nuts (hazelnuts, pistachios, almonds, or a mix)

Lunch Greek pasta salad (whole-grain pasta with red onion, tomato, Kalamata olives, and feta) served on a bed of romaine

Snack Fruit salad

Dinner Leftover seafood stew from dinner on day 11

Day 14

Breakfast Coffee or tea and oatmeal with nut butter and blueberries

Snack Container of Greek yogurt

Lunch Salmon salad sandwich with a cup of bean-based soup

Snack Smashed avocado on whole-grain crackers

Dinner Shakshuka (baked eggs in tomato sauce) topped with feta and served over polenta

Bonus Idea

Breakfast Coffee or tea and toasted whole-grain bread topped with ricotta and sliced fruit

Snack Dried cranberries and mixed nuts

Lunch Quinoa bowl with roasted sweet potatoes, goat cheese, and walnuts

Snack Olives and a few pita chips dipped in hummus

Dinner Artichoke and cannellini bean pasta with bread crumbs and Parmesan

Rich in fruits, vegetables, healthy grains, low-fat dairy, and lean protein, the DASH diet is low in salt. DASH stands for Dietary Approaches to Stop Hypertension. Originally, the diet was designed to help decrease hypertension, but it's a healthy method of weight loss as well.

How It Works

Eating healthful foods is made easier with the DASH diet. This goes beyond a conventional low-salt diet. Foods rich in calcium, potassium, magnesium, and fiber are emphasized in the DASH diet because these nutrients work together to decrease blood pressure.

When following the DASH diet, you should consume lots of:

- Fruit and non-starchy veggies
- You consume reasonable amounts of:
- low-fat or fat-free dairy products
- whole grains
- Lean meats, chicken, lentils, beans, soy products, eggs, and egg substitutes
- Fish
- Seeds and nuts
- Heart-healthy fats found in avocados and canola and olive oils

It's best to limit:

- Sweets and drinks with added sugar
- foods heavy in saturated fats, including most packaged snacks, fatty meals, full-fat dairy, and tropical oils
- Use of alcohol

You can determine how many calories you need to

consume each day with the assistance of your healthcare physician. Your age, gender, degree of activity, underlying medical issues, and whether or not you're trying to maintain or reduce weight all affect how many calories you require.

You can adhere to a diet that permits you to consume 1,500 mg or 2,300 mg of salt (sodium) daily.

When adhering to the DASH diet, you ought to restrict your intake of the following foods:

- foods seasoned with salt
- drinks sweetened with sugar
- meals heavy in saturated fats, like deep-fried dishes and whole-fat dairy products
- packaged foods, which are frequently heavy in sugar, fat, and salt

Consult your provider before adding more potassium to your diet or using salt substitutes, which frequently contain potassium. People with kidney issues or those on specific medications need to watch how much potassium they eat.

Exercise

DASH suggests exercising for at least half an hour per day, most days of the week. The key is to engage in moderately intense exercises for a minimum of two hours and thirty minutes a week. Engage in heart-pumping workouts. Spend 60 minutes a day exercising to help avoid weight gain.

Health Advantages

Numerous studies have examined the many health advantages of the DASH diet. This eating plan may be helpful to follow to:

- Reduce elevated blood pressure
- Lower your chance of stroke, heart failure, and heart disease
- assist in preventing or managing type 2

diabetes
- lower cholesterol levels
- Lower the likelihood of kidney stones

In developing the DASH diet, the National Heart, Blood, and Lung Institute contributed. Additionally, it is advised by The Heart Association of America

You will get all the nutrients you require if you stick to this diet. It is secure for both kids and adults. It is a fiber-rich eating approach that is low in saturated fat and advised for all individuals.

It is a good idea to discuss any health conditions you may have with your provider before beginning this or any other weight loss eating plan.

You will probably be eating a lot more fruits, veggies, and whole grains when following the DASH diet eating plan. These foods are high in fiber, and consuming too much fiber too soon might lead to gastrointestinal distress. Increase your daily intake of fiber gradually, and make sure you're getting enough water.

The diet is generally simple to stick to and ought to satisfy you. It's possible that purchasing more fruits and vegetables than previously will result in higher costs compared to prepared meals.

You can follow the diet if you're gluten-free, vegetarian, or vegan.

Where to Look for Further Details

Visit the "What Is the DASH Eating Plan?" page of the National Heart, Blood, and Lung Institute to get started. – www.nhlbi.nih.gov/health-topics/dash-eating-plan

Books with recipes and advice on the DASH diet are also available for purchase.

There is also the DASH diet for hypertension and the DASH diet for blood pressure.

A plant-forward, semi-vegetarian diet is the general definition of the flexitarian diet.

More precisely, a flexitarian diet is a flexible eating pattern that promotes the consumption of meat less frequently and/or in smaller amounts, integrates dairy and eggs, and stresses the addition of plant or plant-based foods and beverages.

A flexitarian diet has no predetermined macronutrient or calorie targets.

The flexitarian diet's tenets are in line with the 2020–2025 Dietary Guidelines for Americans.

According to new research, adopting a flexitarian diet may help manage weight and lower the risk of diabetes, heart disease, and some types of cancer.

The Fundamentals

The majority of Americans do not get enough dairy, fruits, vegetables, whole grains, seafood, legumes (such as chickpeas, lentils, and beans, including soy), or legumes. A "flexitarian diet" aims to make dietary choices easier by emphasizing what can be added to the diet rather than what should be eliminated, even though a complete diet overhaul may seem daunting.

The combination of the terms "flexible" and "vegetarian" is the flexitarian diet. The term "flexitarian diet" refers to a semi-vegetarian, plant-forward diet that includes dairy and eggs and occasionally permits meat consumption, despite the lack of a universally accepted definition. Without necessitating adherence to the strict dietary guidelines of 100% vegetarian or vegan diets, the emphasis on plant foods is believed to contribute to the health benefits associated with a vegetarian diet.

A flexitarian diet has no predetermined macronutrient

or calorie targets. Rather, the objective is to gradually increase the intake of plant-based or plant-derived foods; meat is still allowed; it is just to be consumed less frequently and/or in smaller amounts.

The majority of the calories in a flexitarian diet are derived from nutrient-dense foods like fruits, vegetables, whole grains, and legumes. Plant-based foods (such as foods made from soy, legumes, nuts, and seeds) are the main source of protein. Dairy products and eggs are good sources of protein; meat, particularly red and processed meats, provides less of it. Owing to its focus on foods high in nutrients, the flexitarian diet promotes reducing intake of sodium, added sugars, and saturated fat.

Your Health and the Flexitarian Diet

Although less strict than a vegan or 100% vegetarian diet, a flexitarian diet can still be beneficial to health. The 2020–2025 Dietary Guidelines for Americans, which advocate choosing comparatively less red and processed meats, sugar-sweetened foods and beverages, and refined grains and more nutrient-dense foods and beverages (fruits, vegetables, legumes, whole grains, low-fat dairy, lean proteins, and healthy fats), are in line with the plant-forward philosophy of a flexitarian diet.3.

A 2016 review of the evidence-based literature looked at the effects of switching to a flexitarian diet and included 25 studies (21 observational studies and 4 randomized controlled trials). Note that the definitions of the diets included in this review varied slightly: from "a diet recommending moderate levels of animal intake" to "a diet comprised of a total of red meat or poultry ≥1 time/month but all meats combined (including fish) <1 time/week and eggs/dairy in any amount." The review discussed new data that points to the flexitarian diet as a potential means of lowering blood pressure, improving metabolic health indicators, and lowering the risk of type 2 diabetes. A semi-vegetarian or flexitarian diet may also be helpful in the management of inflammatory bowel conditions like Crohn's disease, according to the same review.

The flexitarian diet's emphasis on foods high in mono- and polyunsaturated fatty acids, omega-3 fatty acids, antioxidant vitamins, minerals, phytochemicals, fiber, and protein is thought to be responsible for the foods' protective effects.

A growing amount of research is looking at how flexitarian diets can affect heart disease, diabetes, cancer, and weight management, among other health issues.

Heart Conditions

A flexitarian or semi-vegetarian diet that increases the intake of plant-based foods may lower the risk of cardiovascular disease. A diet high in plant-based foods, such as fruits, vegetables, legumes, nuts, and whole grains, has been linked to a lower risk of cardiovascular disease (CVD), according to research.

Diabetes

Numerous studies have looked at the effects of plant-based diets on the risks associated with diabetes. Flexitarian diets are linked to significantly lower insulin, glucose, and insulin resistance levels compared to non-vegetarian diets. They also lower the risk of developing diabetes mellitus.

Cancer

Dietary patterns that are flexitarian or semi-vegetarian have been linked to a lower risk of developing some cancers, including colon cancer.10.

Control of Weight

A flexitarian diet that includes more plant-based foods

may help with weight control. According to research, people who follow a flexitarian diet have significantly lower body fat percentages and body weights than people who follow non-vegetarian eating patterns.

Additional Advantages of Dietary Fiber Sources

Just around 5% of Americans meet the recommended daily intake of dietary fiber, which is 14 grams per 1,000 calories. The majority of Americans only consume about half of this recommended amount. A person's daily intake of dietary fiber, which is important for gut and bowel health and facilitates proper digestion and nutrient absorption, can be increased by eating more plant-based foods. In addition, dietary fiber intake has been connected to a number of possible health advantages, such as a lower risk of hypertension, stroke, coronary heart disease, cardiovascular disease, obesity, certain gastrointestinal disorders, metabolic dysfunctions like type 2 diabetes and prediabetes, and certain cancers.

Sources of Vitamins and Minerals through Diet

Numerous health-promoting vitamins and minerals, such as folate, potassium, phosphorus, magnesium, and manganese, as well as vitamins A, C, E, and K, are found in plant-based diets. These nutrients are essential for the proper functioning of our immune systems, muscles, heart, nerves, skin, gut, brain, and eyes. Frequently, they are not ingested in sufficient quantities. Although the focus of this diet is primarily on the health benefits of plant-based foods, dairy and eggs are also permitted and offer additional nutrients and high-quality protein. Eggs provide vitamins A, D, E, choline, iron, lutein, and folate; dairy contains B vitamins, potassium, calcium, and vitamin D.

Effects on the Environment

Aside from the obvious health benefits, switching to plant-based diets from animal sources can also have a less harmful effect on the environment. When compared to omnivorous diets or animal foods, plant-based foods can help consumers meet functional and nutritional requirements while producing fewer greenhouse gas emissions.

It's important to keep in mind, though, that these comparisons do not take into consideration the reduced bioavailability of some nutrients, like iron and protein, in specific plant-based diets. This indicates that some nutrients found in some plant foods are not absorbed by our bodies as well as they can by our bodies from animal foods. Therefore, when nutrient density is taken into account, the environmental footprints of some plant-based foods do indeed increase.

Ways to Initiate a Flexitarian Dining Plan

Arrange fruits, vegetables, whole grains, legumes, and healthy fats on your plate at every meal.

The majority of the time, choose plant-based foods (such as legumes, nuts, and seeds), dairy products, and eggs when selecting your protein sources.

Enjoy the flexibility of this plan; meat can be added occasionally; just watch the amount that you eat.

Incorporate a greater amount of whole, nutrient-dense foods into your diet, as this may help you eat fewer foods and drinks that are heavy in calories, saturated fat, added sugars, and salt.

To sum up

Fundamentally, the flexitarian diet promotes flexibility, which may be appealing to those seeking a less regimented approach to better health. This diet's primary goal is to gradually increase a person's intake of plants without cutting out animal products. The flexitarian diet, which places a strong emphasis on plant-based and vitamin-, mineral-, and fiber-rich foods, has been linked to a lower risk of type 2 diabetes, cardiovascular disease, and cancer.

The MIND diet, also known as the Mediterranean-DASH Diet Intervention for Neurodegenerative Delay, focuses on the condition of the aging brain. Given that dementia is the sixth most common cause of death in the US, many people are looking for strategies to stop cognitive decline. The MIND diet was first published in two papers in 2015 by Dr. Martha Clare Morris and associates at Harvard Chan School of Public Health and Rush University Medical Center. The DASH and Mediterranean diets have previously been linked to the preservation of cognitive function, most likely as a result of their ability to prevent cardiovascular disease, which in turn protects the health of the brain.

The Rush Memory and Aging Project (MAP) study included residents who did not have dementia at the time of enrollment, and the research team followed this group of older adults for up to ten years. They were chosen from among the senior public housing units and more than forty retirement communities in the Chicago region. Over a thousand people underwent two cognitive evaluations and nine years of yearly food questionnaires. In order to identify foods and nutrients that are linked to protection against dementia and cognitive decline, as well as daily serving sizes, a MIND diet score was created. According to the study's findings, fifteen food items were categorized as "brain healthy" or unhealthy. When compared to individuals with the lowest MIND diet scores, those with the highest scores exhibited a noticeably slower rate of cognitive decline. Compared to the DASH or Mediterranean diets alone, the MIND diet had a stronger impact on cognition.

How it Works

The goal of the study was to determine whether the MIND diet, which drew inspiration from the DASH and Mediterranean diets, could stop dementia in its tracks or prevent its onset altogether. All three diets emphasize plant-based foods while limiting consumption of animal products and foods high in saturated fat. The MIND diet suggests limiting five unhealthy foods and including certain "brain healthy" foods.

Among the nutritious foods recommended by the MIND diet guidelines* are:

- 3+ servings of whole grains per day
- one or more servings of vegetables per day (not just leafy greens)
- 6 or more servings of leafy green vegetables per week
- 5+ servings of nuts per week
- 4+ bean-based meals a week
- 2+ servings of berries per week
- 2+ poultry-based meals per week
- At least one fish meal per week
- olive oil primarily, if additional fat is used

The unhealthy foods, which contain more trans and saturated fat, consist of:

- fewer than five servings of pastries and sweets per week
- fewer than four servings of red meat per week (including products made from beef, pork, and lamb).
- A weekly serving of cheese and fried foods that is less than one
- Less than one tablespoon of butter or stick margarine per day *Note: small amounts of these foods have been used in later research.

Is there alcohol in the MIND diet?

Within the MIND diet score, wine was one of the original 15 dietary components. It was discovered that a moderate amount of wine was linked to cognitive health. But for "safety" concerns, it was left out of later MIND trials. Because alcohol has such a complex effect on each individual, it is impossible to make general recommendations regarding alcohol consumption. A person's personal and family history can influence the range of benefits and risks associated with alcohol consumption. It is a personal choice that you should discuss with your healthcare provider whether or not to include alcohol.

Thus Far, the Research

Foods high in specific vitamins, carotenoids, and flavonoids are part of the MIND diet, which is thought to protect the brain by lowering inflammation and oxidative stress. The MIND diet focuses on brain health, but because it contains elements of the DASH and Mediterranean diets, which have been demonstrated to reduce the risk of heart disease and diabetes, as well as some cancers, it may also benefit heart health and other conditions.

Study cohorts

Researchers discovered that people with the highest MIND diet scores—which indicate a higher intake of foods on the MIND diet—had a 53% lower rate of Alzheimer's disease. When compared to individuals with the lowest MIND scores, even those with moderate MIND diet scores displayed a 35% lower rate. The results supported the notion that the MIND diet was linked to the preservation of cognitive function even after controlling for variables linked to dementia, such as healthy lifestyle choices, cardiovascular-related illnesses (such as high blood pressure, stroke, diabetes), depression, and obesity.

Even after accounting for participants with a history of stroke and Alzheimer's disease, several other large cohort studies have demonstrated that individuals with higher MIND diet scores compared to those with the lowest scores had better cognitive functioning, larger total brain volume, higher memory scores, lower risk of dementia, and slower cognitive decline.

Clinical Examinations

In 2023, a randomized controlled trial was conducted on 604 adults 65 years of age and above who had a first-degree relative with dementia but were overweight (BMI greater than 25), followed a diet that was not optimal, and showed no signs of cognitive impairment at baseline. While the control group stuck to their regular diet, the intervention group received instruction on how to follow a MIND diet. Throughout the trial, registered dietitians provided guidance to both groups on adhering to their prescribed diets and cutting back on daily calorie intake by 250. The MIND and control groups' members both demonstrated enhanced cognitive performance, according to the authors' findings. While both groups lost roughly 11 pounds, the MIND diet group's diet quality score improved more than the other's. The researchers used magnetic resonance imaging to study alterations in the brain, but their results were similar in all groups. The control group, which had been coached to eat their usual foods but had been taught goal-setting, calorie tracking, and mindful eating techniques, probably improved their diet quality as well, which could have prevented significant changes from being seen between groups. Nutrition experts commenting on this study noted that both groups lost a similar amount of weight, as intended. Moreover, the three-year study period might have been too brief to demonstrate a discernible improvement in cognitive function.

The MIND diet does not slow cognitive aging over a three-year treatment period, according to the study's findings. There is still a lot of curiosity about whether the MIND diet or other diets can slow cognitive aging over longer time periods.

Other Elements

Studies have revealed a strong correlation between lower MIND diet scores and poorer cognitive function and higher levels of poverty and less education.

Possible Difficulties

Since it does not call for following strict meal plans, the MIND diet is adaptable. But it also means that in order to follow the MIND diet's recommended foods, people will have to make their own meal plans and recipes. Those who don't cook might find this difficult. People who go out to dine often might need to set aside some time to go through menus.

The diet plan does not limit the diet to eating only these foods, even though it lists the amounts of foods to include and avoid on a daily and weekly basis. Furthermore, it does not highlight portion sizes, exercise, or meal plans.

In summary

The MIND diet is a potentially beneficial eating plan that combines DASH and Mediterranean dietary patterns, which have both been linked to improved and prevented diabetes and cardiovascular disease, as well as supporting healthy aging. The diet can, if desired, also encourage healthy weight loss when combined with a balanced plate guide. Further research is required to expand the MIND studies in other populations, and it is still unclear whether or not adhering to the MIND diet can slow cognitive aging over longer time periods.

This well-liked weight loss plan—which was named the best weight loss diet in U.S. News & World Reports' annual Best Diets assessment—allows you to eat anything you want, including pasta, cheese, and ice cream. The company, formerly known as Weight Watchers, rebranded itself as WW and unveiled the PersonalPoints initiative.

The fundamental idea of eating what you enjoy is still applicable, but according to the company, the program uses a new system to create a personalized plan for you and helps you make healthier food and lifestyle choices.

After asking you a series of personal questions about your eating and exercise habits, WW creates your plan. After that, it assigns you a daily food budget in points and encourages you to stick to it. (Another name for the points is "PersonalPoints." Prior to now, they were known as "SmartPoints." Based on calories, protein, fiber, saturated and unsaturated fats, and added sugar, each food has a point value.

You are encouraged by the PersonalPoints program to eat foods high in fiber, lean protein, and healthy unsaturated fats. It gently prods you to limit foods high in saturated fat and added sugars.

- Additionally, a customized list of healthier foods that "cost" you no points to eat will be sent to you. These "ZeroPoint" choices consist of items such as:
- Produce and fruits
- Low-fat or fat-free cottage cheese and yogurt
- Whole grains and brown rice
- Guacamole
- Fish and mollusks
- Oatmeal and oats
- Whole-wheat noodles and pasta
- Tempeh and tofu
- Chicken

You can now earn points for your daily budget for the first time. These bonus points are awarded for engaging in healthy activities such as:

- Consuming non-starchy vegetables (such as spinach, broccoli, and carrots)
- Increasing water intake
- Increasing your daily movement or exercise

After that, you'll use the WW app to follow the program. There, you'll be able to monitor your daily meals, water intake, sleep, activity, and weight loss in addition to your PersonalPoints budget. You'll receive advice on how to move more and get better sleep in addition to what to eat. You can also include private coaching sessions and one-on-one meetings if you'd like.

The "myWW" program, which offered three different colored meal plans, has been replaced by PersonalPoints. According to WW, adjustments have been made to point values as a result of the PersonalPoints program's increased consideration of nutritional data. For instance, you now need fewer points for foods higher in fiber and good fats (like almonds and avocados).

What You Can Eat and What You Can't

According to WW, there are no forbidden foods. You just keep a food diary and make an effort to stick to your point budget. It's not necessary to purchase premade meals. Additionally, you can simply combine different foods to fit your preferences and goals.

A PersonalPoints budget that will assist you in reaching your goal weight is created using information about your age, weight, height, and sex, among other things. You can use your points however you like, even to purchase dessert or booze, as long as you don't go over your daily allotment. Bonus: You can bank up to four points per day into your weekly budget if you don't use them all in one day.

WW will help you modify your habits more easily in the long run. It's adaptable enough to fit into any lifestyle or diet. You'll make new eating and habit changes as well as adjust long-standing ones.

The amount of work required will depend on how much you are willing to change and how much you will need to change your habits.

You can anticipate learning how to eat out, shop, and

prepare healthy meals in ways that will help you reach your weight loss goals without sacrificing flavor or having to buy strange foods.

When you sign up, WW PersonalPoints asks you a few questions about your fitness level and then suggests daily and weekly activity goals. As previously mentioned, adding more movement or exercise to your day earns you points that are applied to your weekly budget. You get the most points from strength training or high-intensity workouts, but any kind of movement, including cleaning the house, is beneficial.

Does It Support Preferences or Dietary Restrictions?

If you have dietary restrictions related to fat or salt, or are a vegetarian or vegan, PersonalPoints is made to be sufficiently adaptable for you to adhere to.

What Else You Should Know

Cost. There are three different kinds of plans available: The self-guided "Digital" plan costs $4.84 per week and is available to individuals only. "Digital 360" starts at $4.23 per week and offers more support. Additionally, "Unlimited Workshops + Digital," which costs $5.96 per week and provides more in-person time with a WW coach and group, is available.

For $11.08 per week, you can also receive private coaching from a WW specialist. Through the app's members-only social network and in-person community events and workshops that connect you with WW coaches, guides, and other members, you can find inspiration and guidance.

Does It Work?

One of the most thoroughly studied weight-loss plans out there is WW. Indeed, it can work.

You can lose weight and keep it off with the help of this plan, according to numerous studies.

For example, a study published in The American Journal

of Medicine found that individuals who participated in WW lost more weight than those who made independent weight loss attempts.

According to U.S. News & World Report's 2021 rankings, WW came in first place for both "Best Commercial Diet Plan" and "Best Weight Loss Diet," a tie with the Flexitarian Diet.

All things considered, it's a fantastic, customized program with an emphasis on wellness and forming wholesome habits. Losing weight is merely one aspect of it. The WW program helps you build a supportive network by meeting you where you are in your journey.

Is It Beneficial in Certain Situations?

WW is beneficial to all. It can benefit anyone trying to get healthier, but it is especially beneficial for those with high blood pressure, high cholesterol, diabetes, and even heart disease because of its emphasis on wholesome, low-calorie foods.

Make sure to read the labels of any prepared meals you select because some might be high in sodium.

Consult your physician so they can assess your progress as well. For those who have diabetes, this is especially crucial because their medication may need to be adjusted as they lose weight.

The Last Word

This is a great program if you find it difficult to weigh your food or count calories because it does the work for you. To make it simple to stay on track, the online tool gives each food— including foods from restaurants—a numerical value.

The premade meals and snacks make cooking simple even for those who are not experienced in the kitchen. They provide a quick and simple method of calorie and portion control.

No foods need to be eliminated from your diet, but you will need to control portion sizes in order to reduce your calorie intake.

Because fruits and vegetables are prioritized, the diet is high in fiber, which promotes feeling full. It's also easier to follow the program because it's straightforward. WW's prepared meals are also available at your neighborhood supermarket.

The website of WW is a significant asset. Along with weekly live coaching sessions and online support groups, they provide extensive information on wellness practices, cooking, exercise, dieting, and fitness advice.

To reap the benefits of the extensive program in full, budget a certain amount of money. The health benefits of losing weight and keeping it off are well worth the effort.

A period of total or partial fasting from food is known as intermittent fasting. The number of fast days and calorie allowances for various intermittent fasting techniques vary.

This eating pattern may help with fat loss, improve health, and lengthen life, according to some studies. An intermittent fasting program is said to be simpler to stick to than a conventional diet that restricts calories.

An intermittent fasting pattern does not follow random times; rather, it is based on a predetermined schedule. Nevertheless, every person's experience with intermittent fasting is unique, and different approaches will work for different individuals.

Six techniques for Intermittent Fasting

People will prefer different styles of intermittent fasting, and there are many different approaches.

1. Adopt a 12-hour fast each day

This diet has very easy rules. A person must choose and follow a daily 12-hour window for fasting.

Some researchers claim that a 10- to 16-hour fast can induce the body to release ketones into the bloodstream by converting fat stores into energy. This ought to promote losing weight.

For newcomers, this kind of intermittent fasting plan might be a good choice. This is due to the fact that the person can consume the same amount of calories every day, the fasting window is relatively small, and the majority of the fasting occurs during sleep.

Including the time for sleep in the fasting window is the most straightforward method for completing the 12-hour fast.

One may decide to fast, for instance, from 7 p.m. to 7 a.m. They would be asleep for the majority of the time between having to finish dinner by 7 p.m. and waiting until 7 a.m. to eat breakfast.

2. A sixteen-hour fast

The 16:8 method, also known as the Leangains diet, involves fasting for 16 hours a day and eating for 8 hours during that window.

Males fast 16 hours a day and females fast 14 hours during the 16:8 diet. If you've tried the 12-hour fast before and didn't see any benefits, this kind of intermittent fast might be beneficial.

Typically, during this fast, individuals complete their evening meal by 8 p.m., forgo breakfast the following day, and then eat again at noon.

Even when mice on a high-fat diet consumed the same total number of calories as mice that were free to eat whenever they pleased, restricting the feeding window to eight hours shielded them against obesity, inflammation, diabetes, and liver disease (Trusted Source).

3. Observing a two-day weekly fast

When on a 5:2 diet, individuals consume regular portions of wholesome food for 5 days and cut back on calories on the remaining 2 days.

Males typically consume 600 calories and females 500 during the two days of fasting.

People usually set aside different days of the week for fasting. They might, for instance, eat normally on the other days and fast on Mondays and Thursdays. Between days of fasting, there should be at least one day of non-fasting.

The 5:2 diet, sometimes referred to as the Fast diet, has not received much scientific attention. According to a study 107 women who were overweight or obese, calorie restriction twice a week and continuous calorie restriction produced comparable weight loss.

The study also discovered that participants' insulin sensitivity increased and their insulin levels decreased as a result of this diet.

Research examined the impact of this type of fasting on twenty-three obese women. The women lost 8.0% of their total body fat and 4.8% of their body weight in a single menstrual cycle. After five days of regular eating, these measurements went back to normal for the majority of the women.

4. Fasting on different days

The alternate day fasting plan, which calls for fasting every other day, comes in a few different forms.

While some people who practice alternate-day fasting allow themselves up to 500 calories on fasting days, others must completely abstain from solid foods. People frequently decide to eat as much as they want on feeding days.

One investigation among healthy and overweight adults, alternate-day fasting has been shown to be beneficial for both weight loss and heart health. Over the course of a 12-week period, the researchers discovered that the 32 participants lost an average of 5.2 kilograms (kg), or slightly over 11 pounds (lb).

As an extreme variation of intermittent fasting, alternate day fasting might not be appropriate for novices or people with specific medical conditions. Long-term maintenance of this kind of fasting might also be challenging.

5. One 24-hour fast per week

Eat-Stop-Eat diets, which include going without food for 24 hours at a time, include going without food for one or two days per week. A lot of people fast from lunch to lunch or from breakfast to breakfast.

During the fasting phase of this diet plan, individuals are permitted to consume water, tea, and other calorie-free beverages.

On non-fasting days, people should resume their regular eating schedules. This kind of eating lowers a person's overall calorie intake without limiting the kinds of foods they eat.

It can be difficult to maintain a 24-hour fast; you might experience headaches, irritability, or exhaustion. As the body gets used to the new eating pattern, many people notice that these effects gradually become less severe.

Before committing to a 24-hour fast, people might find it helpful to try a 12- or 16-hour fast.

6. The Warrior Diet

One rather extreme type of intermittent fasting is the Warrior Diet.

The Warrior Diet calls for a single, substantial meal at night and a 20-hour window during which very little—typically just a few servings of raw fruit and vegetables—is consumed. Usually, the window for eating is only four hours long.

This type of fasting might be most beneficial for those who have already experimented with other types of intermittent fasting.

People should make sure they eat plenty of vegetables, proteins, and healthy fats during the four-hour eating period. They ought to contain some carbohydrates as well.

While certain foods can be consumed during the fasting period, following stringent rules about what and when to eat over the long term can be difficult. Furthermore, some people find it difficult to eat a meal this size so close to bedtime.

Additionally, there's a chance that those following this diet won't consume enough fiber or other nutrients. This may worsen immune system and digestive function as well as raise the risk of cancer.

General Advice

Maintaining an intermittent fasting regimen can be difficult.

Those who want to maximize the advantages of intermittent fasting and stay on course may find the following advice helpful:

retaining fluids. Throughout the day, sip on plenty of water and calorie-free beverages like herbal teas. This can assist in making sure you get adequate potassium chloride, sodium, and electrolytes.

putting food out of your mind. On days when you fast, schedule a lot of activities to keep your mind off food, like watching a movie or finishing up some paperwork.

unwinding and sleeping. On days when you are fasting, stay away from intense activities; however, gentle exercise like yoga might be helpful.

counting each and every calorie. Choose nutrient-dense foods high in protein, fiber, and healthy fats during fasting periods, if the chosen plan permits some caloric intake during this time. Beans, lentils, eggs, fish, nuts, avocado, and unprocessed meats are a few examples.

consuming a lot of food. Make sure to choose high-fiber, low-calorie foods like popcorn, raw veggies, and fruits high in water content like melon and grapes.

enhancing flavor without adding calories. Use plenty of garlic, herbs, spices, or vinegar to flavor food. These foods are incredibly flavorful and low in calories, which may help to suppress appetite.

selecting foods high in nutrients after the fasting period. Consuming a diet rich in fiber, vitamins, minerals, and other nutrients can help to prevent nutrient deficiencies and maintain stable blood sugar levels. Additionally helpful for both general health and weight loss is a balanced diet.

Prospects

Intermittent fasting can be done in a variety of ways, and no one strategy is universally effective. The best outcomes will be obtained by individuals who experiment with the different styles to determine which one best fits their tastes and way of life.

Whichever form of intermittent fasting is used, prolonged fasting when the body is unprepared can be harmful.

Not everyone may benefit from these types of dieting. These methods might make someone who is predisposed to disordered eating even more unhealthy in their relationship with food.

Individuals with medical conditions, such as diabetes, ought to consult a physician prior to initiating any type of fasting.

On days when you are not fasting, you must consume a nutritious, well-balanced diet for optimal outcomes. If required, a person can get expert assistance to customize an intermittent fasting schedule and stay clear of traps.

To select the ideal intermediate fasting plan that suits their lifestyle, people should get in touch with a registered dietitian.

The Volumetrics diet was developed by Dr. Barbara Rolls, a nutrition professor at Penn State University, with the intention of creating a dietary approach that emphasizes healthy eating patterns rather than a structured, restrictive diet.

The two main concepts in the Volumetrics book series are "energy density" and "nutrient density" in food. While foods with low energy density have fewer calories per portion, those with high energy density have more calories in each serving. In a similar vein, nutrient-dense foods have high nutrient contents in relation to their calorie count, and they frequently contain little to no added sugar, sodium, or saturated fat.

Eating foods high in nutrients and low in energy, such as fruits, vegetables, whole grains, and low-fat dairy, is emphasized in the Volumetrics diet. On the other hand, it is advised to limit foods that are high in energy density, such as those that have a high content of bad fats or sugar and little moisture. The theory is that the body will feel fuller and still lose weight if you concentrate on eating foods that are higher in water content, essential nutrients like fiber, and fewer calories.

Dietary guidelines for volumetrics

Rather than focusing on avoiding particular foods or food groups, the Volumetrics approach emphasizes choosing what to eat. Based on their energy density, foods are categorized into four groups that aid in meal planning and portion management.

Group 1: Foods such as broth-based soups, nonfat milk, and nonstarchy fruits and vegetables

Group 2: Low-fat meat, legumes, starchy fruits and vegetables, cereal, grains, and low-fat mixed dishes

Group 3: Meat, cheese, pizza, French fries, salad dressing, bread, pretzels, ice cream, and cake.

Group 4: Nuts, butter, oil, cookies, chocolate candies, crackers, and chips

Foods in Group 1 are regarded as "free" foods that can be consumed at any time because they have a very low energy density. From Groups 2 to 4, the energy density rises, so in order to prevent consuming too many calories, foods in these groups require greater portion control. Individual differences will affect portion sizes and which groups are included, but most people follow a similar schedule of three meals and two to three snacks per day. Exact measurements are not necessary for Volumetrics diet followers to monitor progress and spot common patterns; however, they can keep track of their food and drink intake in a food journal. Apart from the dietary component, the Volumetrics diet offers detailed strategies for boosting physical activity to 30 minutes or more on most days of the week—a level recommended by the 2018 Physical Activity Guidelines for Americans.

The Volumetrics diet has the advantage of not listing any foods on a "do not eat" list, allowing individuals to freely select which portions of their overall eating pattern to include high-nutrient foods and beverages.

Creating "room" for certain favorites can help frame calorie-dense indulgences in a healthier way, as some research indicates that the more we restrict a food or food group, the more we want it. In particular, it is advised to eat modest amounts of foods that are thought to be high in energy and health, such as nuts (like almonds and walnuts) and common cooking oils (like canola and olive oil). These foods offer the essential fatty acids that our bodies need to produce energy, absorb vitamins and minerals, and maintain the health of our cells. This diet recognizes the importance of including these foods rather than excluding them completely.

Volumetrics nutrition and well-being

Research supports the use of a low-energy-dense diet to improve appetite control and aid in weight loss, even though further research is needed on the role of energy density in weight management and the prevention of overweight and obesity. As opposed to eliminating entire food groups or imposing stringent limits on food intake, the Volumetrics diet emphasizes whole foods and diet customization, making it a more long-lasting eating pattern than popular, short-lived fad diets.

Additionally, some studies have been conducted on the relationship between energy density and particular health outcomes:

Cardiovascular disease: While there isn't enough data to fully support it, some research points to the possibility that a low-energy, high-protein diet may help with certain risk factors for cardiovascular disease.

Type 2 diabetes: Compared to women who followed a lower energy-dense diet, those who consumed diets higher in energy density had a higher risk of developing type 2 diabetes, according to a large observational study.

Breast cancer: A significant observational study found that postmenopausal breast cancer risk was higher in women who consumed the highest energy-dense diet than in those who consumed the lowest.

Weight loss: Lower-energy-dense diets have been linked to lower body weights in a number of systematic reviews and meta-analyses of observational studies. Diets with less energy density have also been linked to better weight management and maintenance after randomized controlled trials.

The majority of these condition-specific studies have an observational design, which means that unlike randomized controlled trials (RCTs), they are unable to establish a cause and effect relationship—that is, that eating a diet lower in energy density lowers the chance of developing a disease. RCTs have been used to test the effects of energy density on body weight, with encouraging findings. However, in order to completely comprehend the impact of energy density on particular health conditions and in various populations, larger and longer-term RCTs are required.

A group of Mayo Clinic weight-loss specialists developed the Mayo Clinic Diet, a long-term weight-management plan.

The program, which has been updated, is meant to assist you in changing your lifestyle by breaking bad habits and forming new, healthy ones. The objective is to achieve a healthy weight that you can keep for the rest of your life by making small, enjoyable changes.

The Mayo Clinic Diet: Why choose it?

The goal of the Mayo Clinic Diet is to assist you in shedding extra pounds and establishing a lifelong healthy eating pattern.

It centers on modifying your daily schedule by incorporating new behaviors and severing ones that may impact your weight. You can lose weight by adopting simple habits like eating more fruits and vegetables, avoiding eating in front of the TV, and getting 30 minutes of daily physical activity.

Based on the most recent research in behavior modification, the Mayo Clinic Diet will assist you in discovering your inner drive to reduce weight, create realistic goals, and learn how to deal with failure.

The Mayo Clinic Diet may be something you decide to

adopt because you:

Would you like to adhere to a program created by medical experts?

Are you trying to find a diet that goes with your eating habits?

like the concept of having an endless supply of fruits and vegetables

Look for professional advice on how to give up bad lifestyle choices and adopt better ones.

Desire to feel great, lower your risk of illness, and improve your health?

Do not want to count calories or eliminate food groups?

Seek a lifelong program rather than a passing trend or short cut?

Are you trying to find simple tips that will motivate you to eat healthier and move more?

Prior to beginning any weight-loss program, always make sure to consult your healthcare provider, particularly if you have any health issues.

How does it work?

The official weight-loss plan created by Mayo Clinic specialists is called the Mayo Clinic Diet. It is founded on clinical experience and research.

The program's main objectives are consuming scrumptious, healthful foods and getting more exercise. It highlights that making lifestyle changes and forming enduring new habits is the most effective way to permanently lose weight. You can customize this program to fit your unique needs, medical history, and dietary preferences.

Two stages comprise the Mayo Clinic Diet:

Lose It! Your weight loss may accelerate during this two-week phase, allowing you to lose up to 6 to 10 pounds (2.7 to 4.5 kilograms) in a safe and healthy manner. You concentrate on lifestyle choices related to weight during this phase. You gain knowledge on how to create five new healthy habits, break five bad habits, and pick up five more bonus healthy habits. You may experience some immediate benefits from this phase, such as a psychological boost, and you can begin forming crucial habits that will carry over into the diet's subsequent phase.

Enjoy It! This stage is a lifetime strategy for well-being. You gain more knowledge about meal planning, portion sizes, physical activity, exercise, and maintaining healthy habits during this phase. Until you reach your target weight, you might see a consistent weekly weight loss of 1 to 2 pounds (0.5 to 1 kilograms). You can permanently maintain your goal weight with the aid of this phase.

The Mayo Clinic Diet also provides electronic tools, like a weight tracker and a food and exercise journal, to help you stay on track with your weight loss journey.

Prioritize selecting wholesome foods

The Mayo Clinic Diet teaches you how to plan meals and estimate portion sizes, which makes eating healthily simple. You don't have to count calories precisely to follow the program. Rather, you'll consume delicious meals that will fill you up and aid in weight loss.

The Mayo Clinic Healthy Weight Pyramid was created by nutritionists to assist you in choosing foods that are satisfying but low in calories. Every food group on the pyramid places emphasis on making choices that promote health. Because fruits and vegetables are good for you in terms of weight and health, the pyramid recommends eating almost anything you want.

Simple food groups at the base of the pyramid should be consumed in greater proportion than foods at the top, and you should move more.

Boost your level of exercise

The Mayo Clinic Diet offers doable and feasible suggestions for incorporating more exercise and physical activity into your daily routine, along with helping you create a plan that suits your needs.

The program suggests engaging in physical activity for at least half an hour each day, and for added health and weight loss benefits, even more exercise. It offers a walking and resistance exercise regimen that is simple to follow and will help you lose the most weight and improve your mental health. Additionally, it stresses increasing daily mobility by choosing to use the stairs rather than an elevator.

To begin a new physical activity program, see your doctor or other health care provider if you have not been active or if you have a medical condition. Most people are able to start with five- or ten-minute activity sessions and work their way up to longer ones.

What's the usual menu for the day?

Five distinct eating styles are offered at varying calorie levels by the Mayo Clinic Diet. There are plenty of recipes and filling meals available, whether you want to stick to the Mayo Clinic Diet meal plan, are a vegetarian, or prefer the Mediterranean diet.

Presented below is an example of a typical 1,200-calorie-per-day Mediterranean meal plan:

Overnight oats with pears and berries for breakfast

Lunch would be a pesto-glazed Tuscan white bean soup.

Dinner is roast chicken on a sheet pan with tomatoes, onions, and broccolini.

Snack: A banana and one cup of sliced bell peppers

Dessert, what about it? Sweets are allowed, but you can only consume 75 calories per day. To be more realistic, try calculating the calories in your sweets over a seven-day period. On Monday, indulge in dark chocolate or low-fat frozen yogurt; after that, refrain from eating any more sweets for a few days.

What outcomes are there?

During the first two weeks of the Mayo Clinic Diet, you can lose up to 6 to 10 pounds (2.7 to 4.5 kilograms).

Following that, you enter the second phase and keep losing 1 to 2 pounds (0.5 to 1 kilograms) per week until you reach your target weight. You can then stay at your goal weight for the rest of your life by sticking to the lifelong habits you've learned.

Almost any diet plan that limits calories can help most people lose weight, at least temporarily. By altering your lifestyle, learning how to handle setbacks, and making better food choices, the Mayo Clinic Diet aims to help you lose weight permanently.

In general, you can lower your risk of weight-related health issues like diabetes, heart disease, high blood pressure, and sleep apnea by losing weight by adhering to a nutritious, healthful diet like the Mayo Clinic Diet.

Reducing weight can significantly improve any pre-existing conditions you may have, no matter which diet plan you choose.

Furthermore, following the Mayo Clinic Diet's healthy eating habits and consuming a diet high in fruits, vegetables, whole grains, nuts, beans, fish, and healthy fats can help lower your risk of developing certain illnesses.

The goal of the Mayo Clinic Diet is to help you live a longer, happier, healthier life in the long run by making it enjoyable, realistic, sustainable, and positive.

Risks?

For the majority of adults, the Mayo Clinic Diet is generally safe. It does promote an endless supply of fruits and vegetables.

Eating a lot of fruits and vegetables is generally beneficial because they give your body fiber and vital nutrients. However, as your body gets used to this new eating pattern, you might notice slight, transient changes in digestion, like intestinal gas, if you're not used to eating fiber in your diet.

Furthermore, fruit's natural sugar does have an impact on how many carbohydrates you consume, particularly if you eat a lot of it. This could momentarily increase certain blood fats or blood sugar levels. That being said, if you are losing weight, this effect is diminished.

With your doctor, modify the Mayo Clinic Diet to suit your needs if you have diabetes or any other health issues. For instance, individuals with diabetes should, if at all possible, consume more vegetables than fruits. Having a vegetable snack is a better option than just a fruit snack.

You consume more fat and protein and fewer carbohydrates when following a low-carb diet.

Things to Eat When Cutting Carbs

Meat, fish, eggs, cheese, and vegetables that grow above ground are the best foods to consume when following a low-carb diet.

Cutting back on carbohydrates has been shown to benefit irritable bowel syndrome, type 2 diabetes, weight loss, and other conditions.

A low-carb diet restricts the amount of carbohydrates, which are mostly present in bread, pasta, and sugary foods. You eat more vegetables and whole foods high in protein rather than carbohydrates.

Low-carb diets have been linked to improved health markers and weight loss, according to studies. Many doctors recommend these diets, which have been widely used for decades. The best part is that using special products or counting calories is usually not necessary. All you have to do to have a full, nourishing, and satisfying diet is to eat whole foods.

On a low-carb diet, you consume more fat and protein and fewer carbohydrates overall. Another name for this is a ketogenic diet. But not every low-carb diet leads to ketosis.

We've been told for decades that fat is bad for our health. Meanwhile, store shelves were overrun with low-fat "diet" products, many of which were loaded with sugar. When looking back, this was probably a big mistake since it happened at the same time as the obesity epidemic started. Although the widespread availability of low-fat products does not establish a causal relationship, it is evident that the low-fat message did not stop the rise in obesity, and in fact, it may have played a role.

Recent research indicates that there isn't much to be afraid of natural fats. You need not be afraid of fat when following a low-carb diet. Just cut back on the amount of sugar and starches you eat, ensure that your protein intake is sufficient or even high, and consume enough natural fat to enjoy your meals.

A diet low in sugar and starches tends to stabilize blood sugar levels and lower insulin, a hormone that stores fat, which may facilitate the body's burning of stored fat. Furthermore, if you are eating a very low-carb diet, the higher protein intake and the presence of ketones may increase feelings of satiety, which will naturally cause you to eat less and aid in weight loss.

A baseline

Consume: Vegetables growing above ground, meat, fish, eggs, and natural fats (like butter).

Steer clear of: Sugar and starchy foods (such as potatoes, rice, pasta, bread, and beans).

When you're hungry, eat, and when you're full, stop. That is how easy it can be. Weighing or counting calories is not necessary.

Notice: Although a low-carb diet has many substantiated advantages, there is still debate surrounding it. The primary risk relates to drugs, particularly those for diabetes, where dosage adjustments may be necessary. See your doctor about any modifications to your medication regimen and any associated lifestyle adjustments. Entire disclaimer

Which beverages fit well with a low-carb diet? Both tea or coffee and water are ideal. Don't use sweeteners if possible. In tea or coffee, a small amount of milk or cream is acceptable (but watch out for caffe latte!).

The odd glass of wine is acceptable as well.

What you shouldn't eat when following a low-carb diet are foods high in sugar and starch. These foods contain a lot more carbohydrates.

A low-carb diet: how low-carb is it?

The effects on blood sugar and weight may be more pronounced the less carbohydrates you eat. We advise, therefore, that you adhere fairly strictly to the dietary recommendations at first. If you're content with your weight and overall health, you can cautiously experiment with increasing your carbohydrate intake—though many people don't seem to want to.

- 0–20 ketogenic
- modest (20–50)
- lenient 50–100

Often referred to as a keto or ketogenic diet, this is a strict low-carb diet. Although the daily allowance of net carbohydrates is less than 20 grams, the diet is not zero-carb.

Three advantages of a low-carb diet for health

For what reason would you think about cutting back on your carb intake? Numerous possible advantages, validated by scientific research and bolstered by clinical practice, exist, including:

Reduce weight

In order to lose weight, most people start eating fewer carbohydrates. Low-carb diets are at least as effective as other diets, if not more so, according to studies. It is simpler to lose weight on a low-carb diet without feeling hungry or needing to track calories.

A low-carb diet may even cause you to burn more calories than other diets, per recent studies.

Turn type 2 diabetes around

Low-carb diets have the potential to reverse type 2 diabetes by lowering or even normalizing blood sugar levels. As the American Diabetes Association points out, cutting back on carbohydrates at any degree is probably a useful strategy for managing blood sugar.

An appreciative stomach

Low-carbohydrate diets can help soothe an upset stomach and frequently lessen IBS symptoms like gas, bloating, diarrhea, cramps, and pain. There are occasions when reflux, indigestion, and other digestive problems get better.

This occurs typically within the first few days or first week of beginning the diet and is, for some, the best part of going low carb.

Cut down on sugar cravings

Try as you might to eat sweets in "moderation," are you finding it difficult to avoid them? A lot of people do.

Low-carb diets frequently lessen, and occasionally even completely eradicate, sugar cravings.

Bonus advantages

The most commonly mentioned advantages of eating low carbohydrate foods are weight loss, reduced blood sugar, better mental clarity, and a calmer digestive system.

However, some people experience even greater improvements, some of which have the potential to change their lives: reduced blood pressure and other heart disease risk factor improvements, improved skin and less acne, fewer migraines, better mental health symptoms, improved fertility, and more.

It takes some new abilities to make a low-carb diet really easy and fun. For instance, how do you prepare your favorite low-carb breakfasts? How can you consume adequate protein? Where can I find more healthful fats to eat? And what should one consider before dining out?

Here are some useful pointers to get you going.

Morning meal

The best time to eat low-carb is at breakfast. Who doesn't enjoy eggs and bacon? Even better options exist that don't include any eggs, in the unlikely event that you responded "I don't."

Since many people on low-carb diets are less hungry and may not need breakfast, having just a cup of coffee is also a great option. You can save a ton of time by doing this.

Lunches

On a low-carb diet, what should you eat for lunch and dinner? There could be delectable dishes with plenty of meat, fish, poultry, vegetables, and high-fat sauces. Our selection of recipes and meal plans will show you that the options are almost endless.

Replace potatoes with pasta and rice

When you can have cauliflower rice or mash instead of starchy sides, who needs them? In addition, butter-fried green cabbage is delicious!

Dining out

Eating low-carb is totally feasible even when you're out and about, like at restaurants. Merely steer clear of carbohydrates, increase your protein intake, and add flavorful natural fats (like butter or olive oil) to your diet.

With a low-carb diet, you probably won't need to snack as much because you'll probably feel fuller for longer.

But if you're in the mood for something immediately, try some cheese, almonds, cold cuts, or even an egg. There are many wonderful choices.

Do you find it difficult to go without bread? Maybe you don't have to. Just remember that there are high-quality and low-quality low-carb bread options.

How much protein should you eat?

Protein intake on many low-carb diets is also higher than what most people are used to. Setting protein as a top priority in any diet is crucial because a plethora of research indicates that diets richer in protein are advantageous for satiety, weight loss, metabolic health, and muscle maintenance.

How to increase your fat intake while following a low-carb diet

When reducing your carbohydrate intake, fat can be an excellent flavor enhancer and source of calories for energy. But what is the recommended daily intake of fat? A hint: just enough to savor your meal without going overboard in terms of calories.

Avoid "low-carb" junk food and processed low-carb foods

Creatively marketed "low carb" products, such as cakes, cookies, candies, chocolate, pastas, breads, ice cream, and other replacement foods, can entice many people following a low-carb diet.

Sadly, things rarely work out this way, especially when it comes to weight loss. These products frequently have more carbohydrates than their labels indicate and are deficient in important nutrients. Avoiding them completely is advised if at all possible.

Potential side effects on a low carb diet

If you stop eating sugar and starch cold turkey (recommended), you may experience some side effects as your body adjusts. For some people these side effects are mild, while others find the transition more difficult. The symptoms usually last a few days, up to two weeks, and there are ways to minimize them.

Another option is to decrease the intake of carbohydrates slowly, over a few weeks, to minimize side effects. But the "Nike way" (Just Do It) may be the best choice for most people. Removing most sugar and starch often results in several pounds lost on the scale within a few days. Even though it's primarily fluids, motivation can still be greatly enhanced by this.

These are some potential negative consequences of starting a strict low-carb diet abruptly.

The keto flu, also known as the low-carb induction flu

"Induction flu" is the most frequent short-term side effect. That is the reason why some people who start low carb feel bad for several days, even up to a week.

Following are typical symptoms:

- Head Pain
- Tiredness
- wooziness
- emesis
- Sensitivity

These adverse effects quickly go away as your body adjusts and your rate of fat burning rises. Their usual duration is a week or two.

Foods high in carbohydrates may be the main cause of this, as they can cause your body to retain more water. Stopping high-carbohydrate foods will cause your kidneys to lose excess water. Before the body has adjusted, this can cause dehydration and increased sodium loss in the first week, which can lead to the symptoms mentioned above.

Upping your fluid intake and, at the very least, temporarily increasing your salt intake will help minimize the effects of the induction flu. Sipping a cup of broth or bouillon once or twice a day is a good option. As a result, the induction flu is typically minimal or nonexistent.

Other typical problems with low-carb

There are six other fairly common side effects of a low-carb diet in addition to the induction flu. It appears that consuming adequate water and salt can help prevent a lot of them as well.

- thigh cramps
- bloating
- foul breath
- Parietal heartbeats
- Decreased physical output
- lower ability to tolerate alcohol

Less frequent problems

These are uncommon problems that typically only affect a small percentage of people:

- Risk associated with breastfeeding
- Gallstone issues
- transient hair loss
- elevated lipid levels
- Hasta rash
- Gaut

Low-carb discussions

Apart from the mostly temporary negative effects of a low-carb diet, there are a lot of debates, misconceptions, and outright myths that don't hold up under closer inspection. For instance, some people assert that proper brain function requires diet rich in carbohydrates. Well, that is just incorrect.

Why eating fat is okay

Many continue to be afraid of natural fat. However, the entire notion that we should be afraid of fat is actually predicated on subpar research that does not justify such a generalized, overarching conclusion. Many open-minded experts now concur that the risks associated with natural dietary fats have probably been exaggerated, as supported by recent research.

Overweight or obesity affects more than 70% of adult Americans, according to the National Center for Health Statistics. However, only roughly 25% of people engage in the recommended levels of physical activity for both aerobic and muscle-strengthening activities.

Experts and research agree that exercise should be a factor in weight loss plans for the majority of people. The foundational weight loss tactic of creating a calorie deficit—burning more energy than you take in—is exercise, and it's one of the best ways to achieve this when combined with dietary changes.

Why Exercise Is Important for Losing Weight

Exercise has numerous benefits, including lowering the risk of chronic disease and promoting both physical and mental health as well as quality of life. It promotes balance and stability, which helps shield older adults in particular from fractures and falls. And it can speed up weight loss efforts when combined with a balanced diet.

Furthermore, it's typical for weight loss sufferers to attribute part of their weight loss to a decline in muscle mass. Exercise increases the likelihood of fat loss, helps prevent muscle loss, and improves a person's body's capacity to maintain their goal weight once it is reached.

Exercise boosts the body's energy-burning efficiency, which makes it crucial for weight loss. "Exposure to exercise burns calories, but having greater muscle mass also burns calories when at rest," says Lauren Weber, D.O., a board-certified physician in obesity medicine and the founder of Deeply Vital Medical in New York City.

Strength training is a common method of gaining muscle mass, which is metabolically active—that is, it needs energy to function, unlike fat. Strength training enhances bone mineral density, muscle quality, and lean mass, but aerobic exercise promotes heart and vascular health, according to Dr. Weber.

Star fitness trainer Don Saladino is an ambassador for Lumen, a metabolism tracking device, and he claims that combining the two forms of physical activity can increase metabolism efficiency, which is crucial for effective weight loss.

"The objective is to increase your resting metabolic rate (RMR) so that you burn calories rather than storing them as fat," says Saladino. "Everyone has an RMR." "Research indicates that combining resistance training with cardiovascular exercise can increase your resting metabolic rate."

How Much Exercise Is Appropriate for Weight Loss?

According to the Department of Health and Human Services' current recommendations, adults should engage in at least 150 minutes of moderate-intensity physical activity per week, with at least two of those workout sessions including muscle-building exercises. In the meantime, adults who qualify as "highly active" put in more than 300 minutes a week of moderate-intense exercise. According to Dr. Weber, the latter category is probably a more useful objective for someone trying to lose weight.

However, Mary Wing, a certified personal trainer and performance coach for the app Future, advises that if you're new (or even somewhat new) to exercising and trying to figure out a safe amount and intensity of exercise for you, it's probably better to err on the side of caution at first to prevent burnout and avoid injury.

Wing continues, "The best exercises for weight loss

depend largely upon the individual and their capabilities." Once that routine feels doable, think about increasing the intensity and/or duration of exercise. "I would suggest starting out with three 30- to 45-minute total body resistance training sessions that target major muscle groups each week and the remainder of that 150 minutes be some form of low impact exercise," the author advises.

The Greatest Exercises for Weight Loss Suggested by Experts

The answer to the question of which particular exercises are most effective for losing weight is up for debate. One broad response, though, is universally accepted by experts: "whatever workout the individual will do consistently."

Having said that, some exercise regimens are more effective than others at helping people lose weight. To that end, try incorporating some (or all) of the following exercises into your fitness routine.

Muscle Training

"Lifting weights" can refer to any kind of resistance training that promotes muscle growth, despite its negative connotations. It makes no difference if the exercise is done with resistance bands, dumbbells, kettlebells, or even strength-training machines in a gym. It qualifies as resistance training as long as the muscles are challenged by a "load."

In order to optimize your resistance training outcomes, Saladino suggests performing "compound" exercises, which are joint-strengthening exercises that involve multiple joints. According to studies, the body is worked much harder during compound exercises like the traditional squat, deadlift, or chest press than during isolation exercises.

Wing concurs and adds that multi-joint exercises put more strain on the joints and muscles overall, which encourages positive muscle change, and raise heart rate more than isolated exercises. Additionally, they transfer most effectively to daily tasks. One of her favorite exercises to teach clients who are strength training to help them achieve their weight loss goals is the squat-and-press combination.

"It's crucial to concentrate on the kind of weight you lose when trying to reduce weight," advises Wing. It should be more important to concentrate on increasing or preserving lean body mass through resistance training than on merely dropping pounds.

Training with High-Intensity Intervals

Short bursts of intense exercise are interspersed with low-intensity recovery intervals in high-intensity interval training (HIIT). For instance, in an HIIT workout on a treadmill, one could alternate several minutes of easy, slow jogging with 30-second bursts of running or sprinting as fast as possible.

As an incredibly time-efficient form of exercise, HIIT is recognized, even though the actual activity may differ. A typical HIIT session lasts roughly 10 to 30 minutes, and it can actually burn just as many calories as a longer steady-state workout. For individuals who are overweight or obese, it may even have a similar effect on body composition to moderate-intensity continuous training.

Wing advises beginning with a lower-intensity modality and longer rest periods to ease into this style of training. Strive to put in at least 30 seconds of intense work followed by at least 60 seconds of rest. Instead of going all out for a sprint, for instance, start with a gentler run or jog for 30 seconds and walk for 60 to 90 seconds, repeating this interval set multiple times, the expert advises.

Water Exercises

With less strain on the joints, aquatic exercise—which can include anything from swimming to water aerobics—allows people to concentrate on building their muscular strength, flexibility, and cardiovascular endurance. Although almost anyone can benefit from working out in the water, Laura Chevalier, director of fitness and outdoor sports at Canyon Ranch Lenox in Massachusetts, notes that this type of exercise is especially beneficial for those who are obese and/or have joint problems because it allows them to work out without the adverse effects of gravity.

Because water is such a forgiving material, one can exercise vigorously and frequently with only a small portion of the negative effects associated with exercise on land. Additionally, working out in the water challenges the muscles quite well. According to Chevalier, exercising in water provides 12 times more resistance than air in all directions while working both halves of each muscle pair (i.e., the triceps and biceps) equally. You can increase resistance by speeding up your movements. Not to add, a 2019 study published in Sports found that heart rates can drop by almost 15% in the water compared to land-based exercises like running, which can improve heart efficiency.

In order to provide a water workout more challenge, stability, and enjoyment, Chevalier also recommends incorporating tools into aquatic exercise. "For variety, try using a kickboard, a pair of resistance bells, or a noodle," she continues.

Walking

According to Wing, walking is widely regarded as one of the greatest forms of exercise for weight loss because it's a low-cost, low-impact activity suitable for people of all ages and fitness levels.

According to research, walking can lower the risk of heart disease and stroke, improve cardiovascular fitness, and both.

Furthermore, walking, at any pace, can aid in the reduction of visceral body fat, or fat that is stored in the abdominal cavity. In fact, a 2022 study published in Nutrients discovered that walking can reduce total body fat at all speeds, though initially, walking more slowly over longer distances is more beneficial for those who are overweight.

As an initial step, just lace your sneakers. You can effectively support your weight loss journey by going for a walk around the block to get some fresh air, meeting a colleague for a walking meeting, and exploring your local city on foot.

Cycling

Depending on their level of fitness, the average person can burn anywhere from 400 to more than 500 calories per hour while cycling, whether they are riding a stationary bike under instruction or cruising along a road or trail. Furthermore, a broader range of people can participate in it because it's a low-impact type of exercise.

Research indicates that cycling can be a significant factor in reducing fat mass and overall body weight when it comes to weight loss. In fact, a very small study published in the Journal of Sports Medicine and Physical Fitness found that overweight study participants lost an average of 3.2% of their body weight and 5% of their fat mass after participating in three weekly cycling sessions without dietary restrictions over a 12-week period.

A person's blood pressure, lipid profile, body composition, and aerobic capacity may all be enhanced by regular engagement in stationary cycling exercises, according to a recent review of research on the advantages of indoor cycling.

Yoga and Pilates

Yoga and pilates can be helpful fitness tools for weight loss, even though they might not burn as many calories as more strenuous cardio workouts.

Pilates works the core muscles, enhances posture, helps with back pain, and prevents injury with a series of exact, rhythmic, fluid movements and a deep focus on the breath. According to Chevalier, it might also have an effect on lean mass, enhance body composition, and aid in lowering total body weight.

Similar to this, Chevalier notes that yoga incorporates particular poses, breathing exercises, and meditation methods that support balance, aid in calorie burning, and build muscle mass and tone. Regular yoga practice also helps to strengthen and stretch the body, enhance body and breath awareness, calm the mind, and enhance balance.

According to Chevalier, "yoga improves many of the causes of weight gain because it is a holistic mind-body practice that improves physical pain, sleep patterns, and reduces stress, which may lead to an increase in cortisol (which can exacerbate fat retention and weight gain)". According to research, yoga can be particularly useful in lowering abdominal obesity in women.

NEAT

Non-exercise activity thermogenesis (NEAT), though not a traditional form of exercise, is crucial for weight loss because it can make up a large amount of an individual's daily energy expenditure for activities like walking, climbing stairs, cleaning, fidgeting, and standing up from a laying position.

Dr. Weber explains that NEAT is the total energy expenditure of an individual, excluding resistance training and intentional exercise. She goes on to say that NEAT may burn a sizable number of calories, which may aid in weight loss and possibly shield obese individuals from metabolic and cardiovascular issues.

"Using a fidget spinner helps burn calories," says Dr. Weber. In order to increase NEAT, she also advocates "habit stacking," which involves performing squats while brushing your teeth. She goes on to say that even small actions like walking, dancing, and using the stairs can contribute to this total.

Indeed, according to a study published in the Mayo Clinic Proceedings, high-effect NEAT exercises like the ones listed above can cause a person to burn an additional 2,000 calories per day, depending on their body weight and degree of general activity.

How to Find Out More About Working Out to Lose Weight

Consult a healthcare professional before beginning any new physical activity program to determine any potential risks, limitations, or contraindications.

Experts advise making contact with a licensed personal trainer or health coach to establish goals, create a fitness regimen, and acquire the right form and technique for your workouts.

Keep consistency in mind as you embark on your weight loss journey. It's also critical to pay attention to your body and follow its lead when it comes to the exercises that feel the best and are most beneficial for you.

Most people are aware of how challenging it can be to maintain healthy weight loss because they have all lived with excess weight at some point in their lives. However, exercise is generally only as effective as consuming fewer calories than burning them off, and weight loss pills have alarming side effects.

A balanced diet and regular exercise are the keys to healthy, natural weight loss that will help you reach your goals. Integrative medicine's tenets assist various hormones, neurotransmitters, and metabolic processes that are compatible with your unique physiology. You will burn fat more effectively as a result of this. However, nutritional supplements and vitamins can support your overall weight loss efforts.

Do Supplements for Weight Loss Actually Work?

It's reasonable for you to be dubious about utilizing supplements to lose weight. Selecting safe supplements that are backed by functional medicine is crucial.

At any given moment, the body is engaged in hundreds of reactions and metabolic processes. Effective weight loss supplements help the body burn fat, maintain stable energy levels, and enhance the utilization of body fat as fuel.

A number of mechanisms are within our control when selecting the best supplement for weight loss. Berberine, for instance, encourages a healthy response to insulin, which encourages the storage of body fat when it stays elevated.

A few amino acids also spare glucose when fuel sources are broken down, enabling the body to choose to burn fat more easily.

For many chronic snackers, controlling appetite and cravings is crucial. We can use weight-loss ketogenic supplements like collagen peptides, spirulina, or MCT to quell those cravings.

When used appropriately, there is a functional weight loss supplement to support every goal; integrative medicine can help you figure out how to use the best natural dietary supplements for weight loss to help you achieve your objectives.

In addition to helping people lose weight, some of natural supplements also support healthy liver function, normal blood sugar levels, and healthy detoxification!

Natural Supplements for Secure and Successful Loss of Weight

1. Herbal Weight Loss Supplement: Berberine

This bioactive substance belongs to a group of plant

alkaloids that are found in shrubs such as barberry and Oregon grape. In fact, berberine has a long history in Ayurveda and traditional Chinese medicine, making it possibly one of the most potent natural weight loss supplements ever discovered. This extract has gained a lot of attention lately because of its capacity to support normal blood sugar levels and the insulin response, two essential components of weight loss.

In a meta-analysis, berberine was found to be just as successful in preserving normal blood sugar levels as oral medications that lower glucose

Additionally, AMP-activate protein kinase, or AMPK, is an enzyme that is activated by beberine. The body's "metabolic master switch" has been unofficially dubbed this enzyme, and turning it on can have advantages akin to those of exercise.

2. L- or carnosine: A Natural Booster for Metabolism

An amino acid is carnosine. It is often referred to as l-carnosine because that is the form that the body's cells utilise more easily.

It has been demonstrated that carnosine can modify the consequences of metabolic syndrome, a condition that affects almost one in six Americans. Because of the dysregulation of insulin, blood sugar, and inflammatory proteins known as advanced glycation end-products (AGEs), metabolic syndrome can make it challenging to lose weight.

Carnosine supports both your anti-aging efforts and metabolic health by assisting in the modulation of the production of these "AGEs".

The amino acids histidine and beta-alanine are combined by the body to create carnosine. But the protein in the carnosine supplements is rapidly broken down into histidine and beta-alanine when it reaches the stomach.

Because of this, research indicates that beta-alanine

supplements increase muscle carnosine concentrations more effectively than carnosine alone, which improves muscle function particularly during high-intensity exercise.

A clean pre-workout supplement that contains beta-alanine might become your new best friend if you want to push yourself a little more during your workout.

For vegetarian and vegan diets, natural weight-loss supplements like carnosine may be especially important. Compared to diets containing meat, plant-based diets offer little to no carnosine.

3. The Fatty Acids Omega-3

Is inflammation causing you to gain weight? Low-omega-3 diets have been associated with increased inflammation, which in turn causes cells to become less sensitive to insulin. The greater our sensitivity to the signals sent by insulin, the greater our propensity to accumulate body fat.

It is not surprising that doctors practicing conventional medicine and functional medicine both highly recommend fish oil and omega-3s because of their role in not only reducing inflammation but also improving heart, brain, and general cellular function.

4. Suculents

This blue-green algae is rich in vitamins, minerals, and phytonutrients such as tocopherols, phenolic compounds, and antioxidants, making it a natural fat burner. It is among the most effective superfoods available. One study that lasted 12 weeks found that spirulina reduced body fat, inflammation, and appetite. Furthermore, research indicates that it also regulates the generation of oxidative stress caused by excess body fat. This could be one way it promotes a normal inflammatory response.

One of Belly Fix's main ingredients, spirulina, helps to

heal digestion and support a healthy metabolism.

Dr. Taz's EastWestTM Way's Belly Fix includes spirulina as a crucial component to help heal the digestive system and support a normal metabolism.

5. Adenosine Peptides

The most prevalent protein in the body is collagen. Numerous functions are supported by it, including digestive and joint health, skin elasticity, and a healthy appetite.

Its potential benefits for weight loss may stem from its ability to soothe the stomach and reduce hunger. Lyptin, the hormone that makes you feel full, is activated by collagen and other proteins. Your brain receives a signal from leptin that it's time to stop eating.

6. MCTs

MCTs, or medium-chain triglycerides, are not brand-new, but their use as a primary component in blends of high-fat coffee has become increasingly popular. They are a common component of supplements for ketogenic weight loss. MCT proponents vouch for its ability to reduce appetite while simultaneously assisting in boosting brain energy.

Is this even possible? For people who are attempting to lose weight, this particular fat may be worth its weight in gold.

Their unique molecular makeup prevents typical digestion and allows MCTs to passively diffuse directly into the liver. They are subsequently further reduced to free fatty acids. They are then transmitted to the muscles or brain, where they support consistent energy and mental clarity.

Furthermore, after entering the liver, MCTs facilitate the liver's natural utilization of other fatty acids, which increases feelings of fullness and decreases hunger and cravings.

The best thing about MCTs is that if our body doesn't need this kind of fat at the moment, we don't store it. Consequently,

MCTs support healthy energy levels and the body's natural utilization of fat as fuel while assisting in the suppression of cravings.

Belly Fix is a straightforward, all-inclusive digestive health supplement that includes coconut MCTs, collagen peptides, and superfood spirulina to aid in digestion, support a healthy metabolism, and encourage the appropriate burning of body fat for energy.

7. Probiotics

One of the many metabolic processes that are dependent on healthy gut bacteria is healthy weight loss. Research comparing the intestinal flora of obese people to those at a healthy weight has revealed a decrease in both the quantity and kind of these beneficial bacteria.

8. B Complex

B vitamins supply some of the most important nutrients for the body, which can be the most difficult to obtain through diets, for a healthy liver and weight loss. They serve a variety of purposes and promote a strong and healthy metabolism.

There are eight distinct B vitamins, and when they are combined in the right ratios, they work best together, or synergistically. The following B vitamins combine to form a B complex:

- (thiamine) in B1
- B2 (pyridoxal)
- B3, or niacin
- PANTOTHENIC ACID, or B5,
- B6 (pyridoxal-5-phosphate, also known as pyridoxine)
- B7, or biotin
- B12.

• Acetate

The body uses vitamin B1 to process carbs into energy. On the other hand, B6 is necessary for controlling the adrenal glands' reaction to stress as well as for promoting blood flow, metabolism, and mobility. B12 is required not only for energy expenditure but also for numerous metabolic processes.

When adding B vitamins, it's critical to choose sources that are fully methylated and devoid of coloring or additives.

9. Verdant

We frequently ignore the liver, which is the hardest-working organ in the body and the foundation of a healthy weight, when attempting to lose weight. It aids in the healthy operation of our metabolism and prevents harmful substances from entering our bodies.

Most people don't realize that a healthy weight AND optimal well-being are closely related to your liver.

Any vegetable in the cruciferous family, including leeks, cabbage, cauliflower, and broccoli, can support the body's natural detoxification processes, which are essential to a healthy metabolism. For comparable advantages, you can also choose any green vegetable with a deep color.

If these foods aren't abundant in your diet, taking a high-quality greens supplement can help you reach your weight loss objectives. In addition, it can support normal blood sugar levels, healthy insulin function, and detoxification pathways.

10. Sleep

Generally speaking, rest is not considered a supplement. Nevertheless, if you're trying to lose weight in a safe and healthy way, getting enough sleep is too crucial to ignore.

Your body is a perfectly calibrated system of chemical messengers and hormones that regulate every aspect of your life, including hunger.

What role does sleep play in the hormones that regulate hunger? Lack of sleep causes our levels of the hunger hormone leptin to rise and our levels of the fullness hormone ghrelin to fall.

This means that while you might be able to tolerate a few sleep-deprived nights, prolonged deprivation will probably cause you to crave high-sugar, high-carb foods that will cause you to gain weight quickly.

Additional Useful Weight Loss Advice

When attempting to lose weight, even small amounts, there are many common issues that we ALL encounter. However, for every similarity we possess, there are an equal number of distinctive characteristics that distinguish us from our neighbors. It is possible that what suits you won't suit any of your friends or relatives, and vice versa.

However, no one solution works well for long-term, sustainable weight loss. Supplementing natural vitamins and other supplements:

Keep an eye on the variety of nutrients in your diet and the portions you are eating. Prior to using the dietary supplements we've listed, try to get important vitamins for weight loss through your diet in addition to adopting a less-is-more philosophy.

Consider incorporating green tea. Although polyphenols and caffeine are frequently found in concentrated form in weight loss pills, their combination produces heat, which increases your body's burning of calories.

Remember that soluble fiber also has the ability to regulate ghrelin and your hunger.

Make a diet change to include more protein because it helps to support your muscles and can help you control your appetite. More muscle mass generally results in increased calorie burning.

Exercise in addition to any natural weight loss supplements to establish a calorie deficit and expedite your attempts to shed the extra pounds from your body.

Working with a functional medicine provider or health coach is crucial in light of these factors. Together, you'll determine which physiologic features complement which weight-loss strategies the best.

Everybody's cause of weight gain is different, so it's critical to find and address any internal imbalances that can lead to both optimal whole-body wellness and weight loss.

You have undoubtedly heard a lot of crazy weight loss advice over the years, such as replacing meals with "cookies" or drinking celery juice every day. These tips are frequently promoted by people who aren't very knowledgeable about health, so if it sounds too good to be true, it probably is. However, for those who are in the right mental health space and have weight loss as a personal goal, there are plenty of valid, research-backed, and expert-approved recommendations out there as well as a ton of misguided weight loss advice that should be avoided.

Making dietary improvements is one such suggestion. According to a study published in February 2023 in Nutrición Hospitalaria, researchers examined data from over 15,000 individuals and discovered that those who consumed the fewest processed foods had a lower risk of obesity, while those who ate the most had an elevated risk. There is a lot of research on the benefits of plant-based diets. Results of a study involving over 200 dieters showed that those who followed a plant-based, low-fat diet for 16 weeks lost significantly more weight than the control group. The study was published in October 2022 in the journal Obesity Science & Practice.

Numerous studies have also indicated that having strong social support—from friends, family, a coach, or even an app or online community—can be beneficial when trying to lose weight. An online support group can help boost motivation, according to research that was published in Digital Health in July 2022. A study published in June 2022 in the Review of Communication Research also concluded that social support is associated with better adherence to weight loss behaviors, based on a 10-year review of literature on the topic of social support in online obesity health communities.

You should also consider your mentality when trying to lose weight. According to research that was published in the journal Obesity in February 2022, people who successfully lost weight accepted their setbacks and saw them as brief interruptions in their plan rather than as signs of failure.

Eat Slowly

We don't always realize when we're full. In addition to enhancing our enjoyment of food, eating slowly improves our ability to recognize when we are full.

Savor Your Food

We're often told what to eat, so when we don't enjoy a particular food, we're less likely to form enduring healthy eating habits. Give new fruits and veggies a try. Learn how to make new, flavorful dishes that offer variety. Spices and herbs can enhance flavor. Alternatively, relish the richness of raw and steamed vegetables and the sweetness of fruit. It's not impossible to have a happy relationship with food.

Maintain a Daily Note of Gratitude

Whether we are aware of it or not, there are instances

when our eating habits and our emotions are related. We might turn to food as a coping mechanism when we're stressed. I help clients practice gratitude by having them write in a journal on a daily basis, or even just when they're feeling stressed. This way, when stress arises, they can recognize it and find other ways to deal with it instead of turning to food as a coping mechanism.

Prep and Cook in Bulk

For example, you can cook a big batch of chicken on Sundays to last the entire week.

Remember the Weights

Make sure you perform two or three weightlifting sessions per week. Increasing your muscle mass can be achieved by using moderate to heavy weights – three or four sets of 10 to 15 repetitions with weights that are challenging for you. Food is more likely to be used as fuel rather than stored as fat when you have more muscle in your body.

Summon Enough Z's

Lack of sleep can lead to weight gain because it raises the hunger hormone ghrelin and lowers the satisfaction hormone leptin. We crave more sweet and salty foods when we don't get enough sleep. For what reason? Because your cravings for foods higher in energy, or calories, intensify whenever you experience greater hunger. Inadequate sleep is also known to impact our ability to think clearly and manage our emotions, so it's not difficult to draw the connection between this and a reduced capacity to make rational decisions in a variety of life domains, including eating. If we were to flip the coin, we could reasonably conclude that our bodies function better when we are well-rested. That would imply that we would only eat until we were fully satisfied when it came to eating. Because our bodies had the time to rest, heal, and rejuvenate, our hormones will also be more balanced.

Never Miss a Meal

Keep in mind that staying alive is our bodies' primary objective. Our bodies literally need calories for life, so as soon as they are denied us, they will take action to survive. Foods with a higher energy density are recognized by our bodies, and we will crave them more. Let your body know when it is hungry, but don't let it believe it is starving. This contradicts a lot of diet strategies, but those strategies don't really benefit people in the long run. Generally speaking, I advise eating every four hours.

Remain Hydrated

Those who drank two glasses of water before meals lost more weight than those who didn't, and they kept it off, according to research. This easy tip has two functions. Anger can be confused with thirst, leading to overindulgence in food. Moreover, drinking water during a meal helps you feel fuller.

Trim Calories, Not Taste

Options like sharp cheddar over mild cheddar allow you to use less while maintaining flavor without making you feel like you're on a diet.

Sort Your Plate Again

Divide your plate in half for vegetables, quarter for whole grains, and quarter for lean protein. You'll notice a difference when you rearrange the portions of vegetables and grains on your plate. With that said, potatoes, corn, and peas belong in the grains category because they are starchy vegetables.

Take it one step at a time, wherever you are

Refrain from feeling as though you must make drastic changes to your entire life right now. Determine your current situation and your desired future state after that. Purchasing a step counter and measuring your daily walking distance is an excellent place to start for individuals who lead mostly sedentary lives. Next, aim for a step goal that is marginally above average and gradually increase it to a daily target of 10,000 steps.

Consider Large, Not Small

Pay attention to the 'big rocks' of weight loss – there are a few areas where you will get the best value for your money. Putting those first and letting go of everything small that adds up to stress will make achieving your goals seem easier and more manageable. Regarding nutrition, be mindful of the amount of calories, protein, and fiber. Prioritize recovery, daily steps, and strength training when it comes to exercise.

See Past the Scale

Although useful, the scale is not the only factor to consider. Keep a running list of nonscale victories and take regular measurements and photos to help you assess progress that may not show up on the scale. This will assist in maintaining perspective and highlight all the beneficial adjustments you're making to your general way of life and health.

Give Protein a Boost for Breakfast

For breakfast, try to get 15 to 25 grams of protein. Protein helps you feel full because it slows down the breakdown process and reduces hunger hormones. A high-protein breakfast also helps prevent cravings from occurring later in the day. Try eating high-protein frozen waffles with nuts, berries, and a touch of maple syrup, or two eggs with whole-wheat toast and avocado. Pair protein foods with fiber and healthy fats.

Actually, Eat Protein with Every Meal

Eating foods high in protein at every meal, particularly breakfast, can help reduce excess weight. Protein has a beneficial effect on your hunger hormones and slows down the digestive process. Additionally, protein can fend off hunger more effectively than carbs. Quinoa, edamame, beans, seeds, nuts, eggs, yogurt, cheese, tofu, lentil pasta, chicken, fish, and meat are examples of foods high in protein.

Aim to Consume Mostly Whole, Seldom Processed Foods

The reason processed foods taste so good and make us want more is because of the numerous processing stages and additional ingredients. They frequently have high added sugar, fat, and salt content. When people are given unlimited access to ultra-processed foods, research indicates that they may consume up to 500 more calories per day than they would if they were given unprocessed foods.

Limit Your Consumption of High-Glycemic Sweets

How quickly blood sugar rises after consuming a carbohydrate-rich meal is measured by the glycemic index. When high-glycemic carbohydrate foods like white bread and potatoes are consumed, especially when they are consumed alone, blood sugar levels will rise and then quickly fall. You become hungry and want more food as a result of this. While more extensive research is required, preliminary findings indicate a connection. However, high-glycemic foods are not completely forbidden. Working with a registered dietitian-nutritionist can offer customized strategies to help you balance your diet and avoid blood sugar spikes, which can help reduce appetite.

Try Different Fruits for Dessert

Fruits are high in nutrients, such as fiber and antioxidants, and low in calories. Just 10% of Americans are getting enough fruits and vegetables, according to the Centers for Disease Control and Prevention. In addition to helping you fulfill your daily needs, having fruits for dessert will enhance the flavor of your meal. A lot of fruits work well baked, grilled, or sauteed. For instance, grilled peaches with shaved almonds and vanilla yogurt on top are delicious!

Consume Lunch Like a Prince, Dinner Like a Pauper, and

Breakfast Like a King.

It's a multifaceted saying, but generally speaking, you should consume more calories in the morning. According to research that was published in the journal Nutrients in November 2019, participants who were given small breakfasts and large dinners lost a significantly smaller amount of weight than those who were given the opposite schedule. Thus, it is possible that eating smaller meals later in the day will benefit people who wish to reduce weight and enhance their general health. The study's intriguing finding was the timing of dinner consumption. They discovered that eating the larger meal, or main course, after 3 p.m. was linked to difficulties with weight loss. It's crucial to understand that this study does not advocate for a 3 p.m. mealtime for everyone. Individual needs—such as those who are pregnant, nursing, have diabetes, or take medication that requires specific foods—may necessitate the need for extra snacks and food. It is crucial that you consult with a registered dietitian or nutritionist for this reason.

Become a Meal Planner

It will save you time, money, and unnecessary calories in the long run to take five to ten minutes on the weekend to plan your menu for the coming week. Can't decide what to have for supper this evening? It's already on your menu plan, so don't worry. Creating a menu helps you stay organized, keep track of the groceries you need to buy and the ones you already have, and ensures that your plate is balanced. Remember that taking a night off from cooking and preparing a frozen meal or ordering takeout is perfectly acceptable. The advantage is that you'll know in advance that you'll be doing that, which keeps you from scrounging when hunger strikes. Make sure to put the plan in writing as well; this will serve as a constant reminder and increase the likelihood that you will follow it.

Make and follow a grocery list

Make a shopping list, either on paper or on your phone (I use Notes, but there are apps for this as well), as soon as you have your weekly menu planned. Having a list of the things you need to buy at the grocery store will help you avoid wasting food, save time, and avoid buying things that just happen to look good but are unnecessary. Don't shop when you're exhausted or hungry if you want to follow your list. Studies indicate a rise in impetuous conduct during those periods.

Examine Everything in Your Kitchen

You need to have the right supplies and kitchenware on hand in order to prepare nutritious meals. Low-sodium canned beans, canned fish, tomato sauce, whole-grain pasta, quinoa, brown rice, low-sodium stock, low-fat plain yogurt, an assortment of fresh and frozen fruit and vegetables, olive oil, and dried herbs and spices are some basic items I suggest keeping in your pantry, refrigerator, and freezer. These are just a few of the components that can serve as the foundation for a tasty and healthful meal.

Possess the Appropriate Equipment

Similarly, easy, effective, and healthful cooking can be ensured by stocking your kitchen with a variety of useful tools. For instance, I love using a seasoned cast-iron skillet for cooking eggs, sautéing vegetables, and making pancakes because it reduces the amount of oil or butter I need to use to prevent food from sticking. An immersion blender, an Instant Pot, baking sheets, measuring cups, spoons, and a hand juicer are a few more of my favorite kitchen tools. Of course, having a good set of knives is a must for anyone working in the kitchen.

Examine food labels

Making it a habit to open your packages on the other side can help you save money, time, and even calories. Food labels provide you with an accurate picture of what you're actually consuming. It's important to note that calorie content matters when trying to lose weight in a healthy way, so read labels carefully. Make sure you're getting a balance of nutrients in your diet without consuming excessive amounts of sugar, salt, or saturated fat to ensure the value of your meals.

Opt for Super Snacks

It's best to consider your snacks to be little meals. Since we are snacking more than ever, it is best to select healthful snacks, such as Greek yogurt with fruit on top or almond butter with sliced apples or high-fiber cereal. Nutritious snacks can help bridge the gap in your diet and increase feelings of fullness and satisfaction because it can be difficult to get everything you need in one sitting.

CHAPTER 6:
SUPPLEMENTS

A strong immune system can help defend against infections, and taking supplements can be a great way to give it an extra boost. We'll take a deep dive into the world of supplements and how they can help you stay healthy. We'll explore what the immune system is, how it works, and which factors can affect its health. We'll also cover key vitamins, minerals, probiotics, botanicals, and other ingredients that play a crucial role in immune support. Finally, we'll go over some safety considerations and when it's time to talk to a doctor about your immune health.

Understanding the Immune System

The body's defense against pathogens and overall health maintenance is the immune system's primary charge. It comprises innate and adaptive immunity, crucial for a robust immune response. Protection against infections relies on a healthy immune system that recognizes and fights specific pathogens to ensure well-being. White blood cells and other immune system cells play a pivotal role in maintaining overall health.

Role of the Immune System

The body's defense mechanism shields against foreign pathogens, promoting overall health. It identifies and eliminates harmful invaders, crucial for well-being. A robust immune system is vital for combatting viral infections and reaping health benefits. Immune cells are pivotal in maintaining overall health.

Factors Affecting Immune Health

Adequate rest plays a vital role in supporting a strong immune system, contributing to immune function. Engaging in regular physical activity is crucial for overall well-being and immune health. A balanced diet rich in whole grains and a variety of fruits is essential for optimal immune function. Moreover, vitamin D levels significantly impact immune health, playing an essential role in immune system function. Managing stress is equally important, as it can influence immune response and highlights the significance of maintaining a healthy lifestyle.

Key Supplements for Immune Support

Vitamins, such as vitamin C, are crucial for supporting immune function, while minerals, like zinc, play a significant role in aiding immune system function. Probiotics are essential for promoting a healthy gut, which is crucial for overall immune system resilience. Additionally, supplements containing elderberry may aid in boosting immune system resilience and supporting overall health. Omega-3 fatty acids found in supplements also help enhance immune health, further supporting immune function.

Role of Vitamins

Vitamin C, a potent antioxidant, is crucial for immune system health, while vitamin D levels are vital for overall immune function. These vitamins, found in citrus fruits and essential for immune health, play a pivotal role in supporting a healthy immune system. By maintaining adequate levels of vitamins, such as vitamin C, individuals can support their immune system function and overall well-being.

Importance of Minerals

Zinc insufficiency can impact immune health, highlighting the significance of minerals. Minerals, including zinc, are crucial for immune function, bolstering overall well-being. Maintaining adequate zinc levels supports immune health and enhances the resilience of the immune system. Dairy products, abundant in zinc, play a key role in supporting immune health, which is vital for overall well-being. Achieving balanced zinc levels is essential for optimal immune function and overall health.

Efficacy of Probiotics

Probiotics support a healthy gut, vital for immune function, and overall well-being. Their role in promoting immune health is pivotal, contributing to immune system resilience. Additionally, probiotics enhance immune system function, supporting overall health. These benefits emphasize the importance of incorporating probiotics into a daily routine to maintain a healthy immune system.

Breakdown of Essential Vitamins

Vitamin A maintains healthy vision and immune function. Vitamin C acts as a powerful antioxidant, supporting immune system function. Vitamin D aids immune response and overall health, aiding in calcium absorption. These essential vitamins play a critical role in supporting the body's innate immune system, especially during the winter months when physical stress is higher. Incorporating a variety of fruits, orange juice, and healthy eating habits ensures sufficient intake of these vital nutrients.

Vitamin A

Supporting immune function, vitamin A promotes the growth and health of immune cells. Its adequate intake helps maintain skin and respiratory tract integrity, essential for immune response. Foods rich in vitamin A include liver, fish, and dairy products, contributing to a healthy immune system. Vitamin A also aids in maintaining healthy vision and overall immune function.

Vitamin C

Enhancing the function of white blood cells, vitamin C supports the immune system's response to foreign pathogens. Citrus fruits, strawberries, and bell peppers are excellent sources, crucial for immune health. Adequate intake is linked to reduced cold duration and beneficial effects on respiratory infections, making it a vital nutrient during winter months.

Vitamin D

Adequate levels of vitamin D are crucial for maintaining a healthy immune system and reducing the risk of respiratory tract infections. The deficiency of vitamin D is associated with an increased risk of respiratory infections and autoimmune diseases. Sources of vitamin D include sunlight exposure, fatty fish, and fortified foods, all of which play an important role in immune system function.

Significance of Crucial Minerals

Selenium, a potent antioxidant, safeguards cells from free radicals, bolstering immune health. Meanwhile, zinc deficiency can compromise immune function, hindering the body's ability to fight infections. Consuming whole grains, nuts, and seeds can help maintain adequate levels of selenium and zinc, crucial for immune support. Incorporating these minerals through food or supplements can significantly impact immune health, providing vital protection against illnesses.

Selenium

Selenium, an essential mineral, plays a crucial role in immune response by regulating inflammation and supporting immune system function. It can be found in Brazil nuts, seafood, and whole grains, serving as rich sources beneficial for immune health. Deficiency in selenium is associated with an increased risk of viral infections and respiratory tract infections, emphasizing its importance in maintaining a healthy immune system.

Zinc

Supporting the immune system, zinc is crucial for the development and function of immune cells. Adequate zinc intake from foods like oysters, beef, and legumes can aid in maintaining a healthy immune system. Additionally, zinc supplements have shown potential in reducing the duration of colds and supporting overall immune health. Incorporating zinc into your diet or as a supplement could play an important role in supporting human health.

Incorporating Botanicals for Immune Boosting

Echinacea, a traditional immune supporter, may reduce the risk of respiratory infections. Elderberry supplements have shown benefits for cold and flu symptoms, aiding immune function. Integrating botanicals into the diet can contribute to a balanced immune response, enhancing overall immune health. This natural approach offers additional support to the body's innate immune system without introducing physical stress or side effects.

Echinacea

Echinacea, a traditional immune system supporter, modulates immunity, potentially enhancing natural defense mechanisms. Scientific research indicates its potential to reduce respiratory tract infection risk, bolstering immune health. Echinacea supplements aid immune function, protecting against common colds. When used as a part of a healthy diet, echinacea may contribute to balanced immune response, promoting overall well-being.

Elderberry

Elderberry supplements contain compounds that aid immune system function and the body's response to viral infections. Studies indicate that consuming elderberry supplements may reduce flu symptoms' severity and duration, beneficial for immune health. Traditionally used to promote immune health, elderberry offers potential benefits during flu season. The fruit is rich in vitamins C and antioxidants, supporting overall well-being and immune function. Its efficacy and safety make elderberry an essential addition to one's wellness routine.

Role of Other Ingredients in Immune Health

Supplements often include zinc, supporting immune function, while some feature elderberry, known for its immune-boosting properties. Certain supplements may also contain echinacea, believed to enhance immune health. Additionally, omega-3 fatty acids in supplements help regulate immune function, and probiotics aid in maintaining a healthy immune system. These ingredients play an important role in supporting overall immune health and function.

Omega-3 Fatty Acids

Omega-3 fatty acids, found in fish oil and certain nuts, play a crucial role in reducing inflammation and supporting the immune response. These essential fatty acids contribute significantly to overall immune health and function by aiding immune cells in their response to pathogens. Studies suggest that omega-3s may enhance immune function, potentially reducing the risk of infections. By incorporating supplements rich in omega-3 fatty acids, individuals can bolster their immune system's resilience to various health challenges.

How do these supplements enhance your immune system?

Supplements enhance your immune system by providing essential vitamins, minerals, probiotics, and antioxidants. They support optimal immune function, promote a healthy gut, and contribute to a balanced diet necessary for immune health. Omega-3 fatty acids in supplements also play a role in boosting immune resilience.

Safety Considerations

Before incorporating any new supplements, consulting a healthcare professional is crucial. It's essential to research potential side effects, especially if you have existing health conditions, and ensure that the supplements won't interact with any current medications. Additionally, excessive intake of vitamins and minerals should be approached with caution due to potential adverse effects. Opting for supplements from reputable sources can guarantee quality and safety, minimizing potential risks.

When to Talk to a Doctor

If unexpected side effects occur from supplement intake, seek medical advice promptly. Consult a doctor before taking supplements, especially if pregnant or breastfeeding. Discuss any significant health changes after starting supplements with a healthcare professional. Individuals with chronic health issues should obtain clearance from a doctor before supplementing. Seek medical guidance when considering supplements for children as their needs differ from adults.

Conclusion

In conclusion, incorporating supplements into your daily routine can play a significant role in boosting your immune system. Vitamins such as A, C, and D, along with minerals like selenium and zinc, are crucial for maintaining optimal immune health. Probiotics and botanicals like echinacea and elderberry also contribute to strengthening your body's defenses. However, it's essential to consider safety considerations and consult with a healthcare professional before starting any new supplement regimen. By taking proactive steps to support your immune system, you can enhance your overall well-being and protect yourself from illnesses. Remember, a healthy immune system is key to leading a vibrant and active life.

CHAPTER 7: STRESS

How Stress Affects Your Immune System

Stress is a part of our daily lives, and it can even be useful at times. However, when stress becomes chronic, it can have a detrimental effect on the immune system. Chronic stress causes an imbalance in the body's natural defense mechanisms, making us more susceptible to infections and illnesses. We will explore the relationship between stress and the immune system in-depth. We'll look at how chronic stress affects immune function, the psychological aspect of stress and its role in immunity, identifying stressors that influence immunity, and the role of lifestyle factors in managing stress and boosting immunity. We will also cover ways to reduce stress for better immunity, including meditation and other relaxation techniques. By understanding how stress affects the immune system, you can take steps to manage your stress levels and improve your overall health.

Understanding the Impact of Stress on the Immune System

Chronic stress can alter the number of natural killer cells, leading to immune dysregulation and systemic inflammation. This can impact immune reactions and potentially hinder the healing process, affecting the body's defensive responses. Psychological stressors influence human health by impacting immune function.

The Basics of Stress and the Immune System

The body's response to acute stress can impact the immune system, affecting disease susceptibility. Stress has the potential to influence immune function, thereby impacting the body's healing processes. Psychological stressors may affect immune cells, subsequently influencing human health. Additionally, exposure to stress has been found to influence immune reactions, potentially impacting overall human health.

How Chronic Stress Affects Immune Function

Chronic stress exposure can impact immune function, affecting human health. This may influence disease susceptibility as well as tissue damage and the healing process. Immune cells are particularly vulnerable to chronic stress, potentially leading to compromised immune reactions. The function of the immune system is intricately linked to chronic stress levels and can significantly affect overall human health.

The Psychological Aspect of Stress and Its Role in Immunity

Psychological stressors have the potential to influence immune response and impact human health. The effects of stress on immune function can potentially affect tissue damage and the healing process. Stress exposure is linked to varied immune reactions, which may ultimately impact human health and disease susceptibility. Furthermore, stress can alter immune system function, influencing the body's ability to fight off diseases. Moreover, psychological stress can also influence immune cells, potentially impacting overall human health and well-being.

The Mind-Body Connection: Stress and Immunity

The link between the mind and body greatly impacts immune function, potentially influencing overall human health. Psychological stressors have the ability to affect immune response, which can impact tissue damage and the healing process. Exposure to stress has the potential to influence immune reactions, which in turn can affect human health. Additionally, immune cells may be influenced by psychological stress, further impacting human health and well-being. The intricate connection between the mind and body plays a significant role in determining the body's ability to combat diseases and maintain overall health.

Coping Mechanisms and Their Impact on the Immune System

Implementing effective coping mechanisms has the potential to alleviate the impact of stress on immune function. Mind-body practices such as meditation are believed to have a modulating effect on the influence of stress on immune function. Additionally, social support can act as a buffer against the adverse effects of stress on immune function, thereby promoting overall health. Making healthy lifestyle choices is also crucial in supporting immune function and possibly mitigating the effects of stress. Furthermore, coping strategies may play a significant role in influencing immune response, thus potentially impacting disease susceptibility.

Identifying Stressors and Their Influence on Immunity

Chronic stress can impact immune reactions, potentially affecting human health. Stress exposure influences immune response, potentially impacting tissue damage and the healing process. Moreover, psychological stressors can influence immune system function, potentially impacting disease susceptibility and overall health. Additionally, stressed mice have shown changes in their gut microbiota, which can further impact immune response. Recent work also suggests that stress can influence white blood cells and T cells, affecting the body's ability to fight off infections and diseases. These findings emphasize the intricate relationship between stress and the immune system, warranting further research for comprehensive understanding.

Everyday Stressors and Immune Response

Impactful daily stressors can influence immune function, potentially affecting disease susceptibility. Psychological stressors have the potential to impact immune response, influencing human health. Stress's effect on immune system function may influence tissue damage and the healing process. Exposure to stress can potentially impact immune reactions, affecting human health. Stress exposure may also impact the body's ability to fight off diseases.

Major Life Events and Their Effect on Immunity

When major life events occur, they can influence immune response, potentially impacting human health. The effect of stress on immune function may impact tissue damage and the healing process. Stress exposure has the potential to impact immune reactions, thereby affecting human health. Psychological stress may also influence immune cells, which in turn could impact human health. Ultimately, stress affects immune system function, potentially impacting disease susceptibility. All these factors highlight the intricate connection between major life events, stress, and the immune system, shedding light on the profound impact of stress on human health.

The Role of Lifestyle Factors in Stress Management and Immunity

Healthy lifestyle choices support immune function, possibly mitigating stress effects. Diet and exercise may modulate stress impact on immunity. Regular physical activity can positively impact immune function, potentially mitigating stress. Proper nutrition supports immune function, potentially alleviating stress effects. Lifestyle choices influence immune response, potentially impacting disease susceptibility.

Importance of Diet and Exercise in Stress Management

Incorporating a well-balanced diet and regular exercise routine is crucial in managing chronic stress and supporting immune function. Poor dietary choices and sedentary lifestyle can contribute to chronic stress, leading to weakened immunity. Consuming nutrient-rich foods can help reduce stress levels and promote optimal immune health. Similarly, engaging in regular physical activity can effectively lower stress levels and enhance immune function. Additionally, relaxation techniques such as meditation and yoga play a vital role in stress management and immune support. Prioritizing self-care practices is essential for overall health and wellbeing during times of heightened stress.

Sleep and Its Role in Managing Stress

Sleep plays a vital role in stress management and

immune function. Inadequate sleep can elevate stress levels and compromise the immune system's resilience. The body requires sufficient sleep to repair and regenerate, promoting stress reduction and improved immune response. Disrupted sleep patterns and disturbances can exacerbate stress and weaken the immune system. Implementing better sleep strategies, such as establishing a calming bedtime routine and minimizing screen time before sleep, can effectively mitigate stress and enhance immune function. Prioritizing quality sleep is crucial for overall stress management and optimal immune health.

Ways to Reduce Stress for Better Immunity

Chronic stress weakens the immune system, increasing the risk of infections. Stress reduction techniques like meditation and exercise can boost immunity. Adequate sleep and good nutrition strengthen the immune system. Social support and positive relationships reduce stress and improve health. Seeking help from a mental health professional is beneficial for managing stress and improving immunity. Integrating these strategies into daily life can significantly enhance overall well-being and immune function.

Can Regular Meditation Improve Your Immune Response?

Regular meditation can have a positive impact on your immune response. By reducing inflammation and stress levels, it supports immune system function. Incorporating mindfulness techniques into your daily routine can improve mental health and overall well-being, leading to a stronger immune system.

Conclusion

In conclusion, chronic stress can have a detrimental impact on your immune system. It weakens the body's defense mechanisms and makes you more susceptible to illnesses. Understanding the connection between stress and immunity is crucial for maintaining good health. It's important to identify your stressors and find effective ways to manage them. Incorporating stress-reducing activities like meditation, exercise, and proper sleep into your lifestyle can significantly improve your immune response. Take care of your mental well-being and prioritize self-care to strengthen your immune system and protect your overall health. Remember, a healthy mind and body go hand in hand.

If you enjoyed this book, you may also enjoy:

The Serotonin Book: How to Maximize Serotonin Levels Naturally

The Brain Book: How to Maximize the Potential of Your Brain Naturally

The GABA Book: How to Maximize Your Brain's Calming Power Naturally

Follow the author on Instagram for free book giveaways (no strings attached), free mental health information, and more:

@alexander_wright_books

For a complete list of works by this author, visit:

Badfeelingsgoaway.com

References

Nieman, D. C., & Wentz, L. M. (2019, May). The compelling link between physical activity and the body's defense system. *Journal of Sport and Health Science, 8*(3), 201–217. https://doi.org/10.1016/j.jshs.2018.09.009

Sheikh, K. (2022, September 7). *Can Exercise Strengthen Your Immunity?* The New York Times. https://www.nytimes.com/2022/09/07/well/move/exercise-immunity-covid.html

RDN, K. W. (2022, November 16). *Fight off the flu with immune-boosting nutrients.* Mayo Clinic Health System. https://www.mayoclinichealthsystem.org/hometown-health/speaking-of-health/fight-off-the-flu-with-nutrients

What is Noradrenaline? (n.d.). Mental Health America. https://mhanational.org/what-noradrenaline

Histamine Intolerance. (n.d.). Histamine Intolerance: Causes, Symptoms, and Diagnosis. https://www.healthline.com/health/histamine-intolerance

Malík, M., & Tlustoš, P. (2022, August 17). *Nootropics as Cognitive Enhancers: Types, Dosage and Side Effects of Smart Drugs.* PubMed Central (PMC). https://doi.org/10.3390/nu14163367

;Watson NF;Badr MS;Belenky G;Bliwise DL;Buxton OM;Buysse D;Dinges DF;Gangwisch J;Grandner MA;Kushida C;Malhotra RK;Martin JL;Patel SR;Quan SF;Tasali E; ;Twery M;Croft JB;Maher E; ;Barrett JA;Thomas SM;Heald JL; (n.d.). *Recommended amount of sleep for a healthy adult: A joint consensus statement of the American Academy of Sleep Medicine and Sleep Research Society.* Journal of clinical sleep medicine : JCSM : official publication of the American Academy of Sleep Medicine. Retrieved April 18, 2023, from https://pubmed.ncbi.nlm.nih.gov/25979105/

Paruthi S;Brooks LJ;D'Ambrosio C;Hall WA;Kotagal S;Lloyd RM;Malow BA;Maski K;Nichols C;Quan SF;Rosen CL;Troester MM;Wise MS; (n.d.). *Consensus statement of the American Academy of Sleep Medicine on the recommended amount of sleep for Healthy Children: Methodology and discussion.* Journal of clinical sleep medicine : JCSM : official publication of the American Academy of Sleep Medicine. Retrieved April 18, 2023, from https://pubmed.ncbi.nlm.nih.gov/27707447/

Oversleeping: Bad   for   your   health? Oversleeping: Bad for Your Health? | Johns Hopkins Medicine. (2021, October 20). Retrieved April 18, 2023, from https://www.hopkinsmedicine.org/health/wellness-and-prevention/oversleeping-bad-for-your-health

U.S. Department of Health and Human Services. (n.d.). *What are sleep deprivation and deficiency?* National Heart Lung and Blood Institute. Retrieved April 18, 2023, from https://www.nhlbi.nih.gov/health/sleep-deprivation#:~:text=Sleep%20deficiency%20is%20linked%20to,adults%2C%20teens%2C%20and%20children.

U.S. Department of Health and Human Services. (n.d.). *How sleep works.* National Heart Lung and Blood Institute. Retrieved April 18, 2023, from https://www.nhlbi.nih.gov/health/sleep/

Vora, E., Ellen Vora As a psychiatrist with an integrative focus, & Vora, E. (2018, November 8). *How to relieve insomnia without medication: Part 1.* One Medical. Retrieved April 18, 2023, from https://www.onemedical.com/blog/get-well/how-to-relieve-insomnia-without-medication-part-1/

Melatonin. Uses, Interactions, Mechanism of Action | DrugBank Online. (n.d.). Retrieved April 18, 2023, from https://go.drugbank.com/drugs/DB01065

Foods that are high in melatonin. The Sleep Doctor. (2023, February 10). Retrieved April 18, 2023, from https://thesleepdoctor.com/melatonin/foods-with-melatonin/

Histamine. Cleveland Clinic. (n.d.). Retrieved April 19, 2023,   from   https://my.clevelandclinic.org/health/articles/24854-histamine

A;, B. A. K. R. K. P.-L. (n.d.). *Learning and memory.* Handbook of clinical neurology. Retrieved April 19, 2023, from https://pubmed.ncbi.nlm.nih.gov/24112934/

Anti-histamine foods. Root Functional Medicine. (2023, January 5). Retrieved April 19, 2023, from https://rootfunctionalmedicine.com/anti-histamine-foods

Foster, J. (2021, September 9). *9 natural antihistamines used to prevent histamine reactions*. SelfDecode Supplements. Retrieved April 19, 2023, from https://supplements.selfdecode.com/blog/natural-antihistamines/

Therapeutic Goods Administration (TGA). (2022, September 27). *First-generation oral sedating antihistamines - do not use in children*. Therapeutic Goods Administration (TGA). Retrieved April 19, 2023, from https://www.tga.gov.au/news/safety-updates/first-generation-oral-sedating-antihistamines-do-not-use-children

Natural sleep aids: Which ones are safe? Sleep Foundation. (2023, April 12). Retrieved April 20, 2023, from https://www.sleepfoundation.org/sleep-aids/natural-sleep-aids

Cognitive behavioral therapy for insomnia (CBT-I). Sleep Foundation. (2023, March 3). Retrieved April 20, 2023, from https://www.sleepfoundation.org/insomnia/treatment/cognitive-behavioral-therapy-insomnia

WebMD. (n.d.). *Side effects of sleeping pills: Common and potentially harmful side effects*. WebMD. Retrieved April 20, 2023, from https://www.webmd.com/sleep-disorders/understanding-the-side-effects-of-sleeping-pills

Tens for sleep aid. Massage Therapy Concepts. (2022, May 2). Retrieved April 20, 2023, from https://massagetherapyconcepts.com/a/blog/tens-for-sleeping

#15: Why sleep science and EMS technology go hand in hand. PowerDot.com. (n.d.). Retrieved April 20, 2023, from https://www.powerdot.com/blogs/training/sleep-science-and-ems#:~:text=You%20can%20improve%20the%20quality,slip

%20into%20more%20restful%20sleep.

National Center for Biotechnology Information. (n.d.). Retrieved April 20, 2023, from https://www.ncbi.nlm.nih.gov/pmc/articles/PMC8254331/

How effective is hypnosis to help you fall asleep? Sleep Foundation. (2022, May 6). Retrieved April 20, 2023, from https://www.sleepfoundation.org/sleep-hypnosis

Essential oils to help you get more sleep. Sleep Foundation. (2022, April 13). Retrieved April 20, 2023, from https://www.sleepfoundation.org/best-essential-oils-for-sleep

WebMD. (n.d.). *Alternative treatments & remedies for insomnia.* WebMD. Retrieved April 20, 2023, from https://www.webmd.com/sleep-disorders/alternative-treatments-for-insomnia

Cortisol: What it is, function, symptoms & levels. Cleveland Clinic. (n.d.). Retrieved April 20, 2023, from https://my.clevelandclinic.org/health/articles/22187-cortisol

12 foods that can help lower cortisol for a healthy body & mind. VEGAMOUR. (n.d.). Retrieved April 20, 2023, from https://vegamour.com/blogs/blog/foods-that-lower-cortisol

Modi, J. (2022, July 13). *Are there supplements to reduce cortisol (stress hormone)?* Buzzrx.com. Retrieved April 20, 2023, from https://www.buzzrx.com/blog/are-there-supplements-to-reduce-cortisol-stress-hormone

Norepinephrine: What it is, function, deficiency & side effects. Cleveland Clinic. (n.d.). Retrieved April 20, 2023, from https://my.clevelandclinic.org/health/articles/22610-norepinephrine-noradrenaline

How to balance adrenaline levels naturally. Rupa Health. (2023, March 2). Retrieved April 20, 2023, from https://www.rupahealth.com/post/adrenaline#:~:text=Eating%20a%20well%2Dbalanced%20diet,can%20help%20balance

%20norepinephrine%20levels.

Hypnogogic hallucinations: Causes, symptoms & treatment. Cleveland Clinic. (n.d.). Retrieved April 20, 2023, from https://my.clevelandclinic.org/health/articles/23234-hypnagogic-hallucinations

WebMD. (n.d.). *Sleep paralysis - causes, symptoms, treatment, and prevention.* WebMD. Retrieved April 20, 2023, from https://www.webmd.com/sleep-disorders/sleep-paralysis

WebMD. (n.d.). *Adult nightmares: Causes and treatments.* WebMD. Retrieved April 20, 2023, from https://www.webmd.com/sleep-disorders/nightmares-in-adults

The Ultimate Gut Health Grocery List for Beginners | Nourish. (2023, June 13). The Ultimate Gut Health Grocery List for Beginners | Nourish. https://www.usenourish.com/blog/gut-health-grocery-list

The Brain-Gut Connection. (2021, November 1). The Brain-Gut Connection | Johns Hopkins Medicine. https://www.hopkinsmedicine.org/health/wellness-and-prevention/the-brain-gut-connection

Ruscio, D. M. (2022, November 21). *Foods that boost serotonin: The impact on Gut & Brain Health.* Dr. Michael Ruscio, DC. Retrieved March 10, 2023, from https://drruscio.com/foods-that-boost-serotonin/

Serotonin: What is it, Function & Levels. Cleveland Clinic. (n.d.). Retrieved March 10, 2023, from https://my.clevelandclinic.org/health/articles/22572-serotonin

Gotter, A. (2018, September 29). *What is tryptophan? uses, benefits, and foods.* Healthline. Retrieved March 14, 2023, from https://www.healthline.com/health/tryptophan#common-uses

Young, S. N. (2007, November). *How to increase serotonin in the human brain without drugs.* Journal of psychiatry &

neuroscience : JPN. Retrieved March 14, 2023, from https://www.ncbi.nlm.nih.gov/pmc/articles/PMC2077351/

Migala, J. (2023, August 16). *Mediterranean Diet: Complete Food List and 14-Day Meal Plan*. EverydayHealth.com. https://www.everydayhealth.com/mediterranean-diet/complete-mediterranean-diet-food-list-day-meal-plan/

Understanding the DASH diet: MedlinePlus Medical Encyclopedia. (n.d.). https://medlineplus.gov/ency/patientinstructions/000784.htm

Rd, A. P. (2021, November 3). *What is the Flexitarian Diet?* Food Insight. https://foodinsight.org/what-is-the-flexitarian-diet/#:~:text=More%20specifically%2C%20the%20flexitarian%20diet,goals%20in%20a%20flexitarian%20diet.

Diet Review: MIND Diet. (2023, August 11). The Nutrition Source. https://www.hsph.harvard.edu/nutritionsource/healthy-weight/diet-reviews/mind-diet/

Health & Diet. (n.d.). WebMD. https://www.webmd.com/diet

Leonard, J. (2023, March 6). *Six ways to do intermittent fasting*. https://www.medicalnewstoday.com/articles/322293

Eenfeldt, A. (2023, March 21). *A low carb diet for beginners*. Diet Doctor. https://www.dietdoctor.com/low-carb

The Mayo Clinic Diet: A weight-loss program for life. (2023, May 4). Mayo Clinic. https://www.mayoclinic.org/healthy-lifestyle/weight-loss/in-depth/mayo-clinic-diet/art-20045460

Insight, F. (2019, June 26). *The Basics of the Volumetrics Diet*. Food Insight. https://foodinsight.org/basics-of-volumetrics-diet/#:~:text=The%20Volumetrics%20diet%20emphasizes%20eating,are%20recommended%20to%20be%20limited.

Rd, R. R. M. (2023, February 22). *The 9 Best Diet Plans for*

Your Overall Health. Healthline. https://www.healthline.com/nutrition/best-diet-plans

Neumann, K. D. (2023, August 16). *7 Best Exercises For Weight Loss, According To Experts*. Forbes Health. https://www.forbes.com/health/fitness/best-exercises-for-weight-loss/

C., & C. (2023, August 16). *Top 10 Best Natural Dietary Supplements for Weight Loss*. CentreSpring MD. https://centrespringmd.com/top-10-best-natural-supplements-for-weight-loss/

Hochwald, L. (2023, April 7). *Lose Weight the Healthy Way with 25 Tips From Registered Dietitians*. EverydayHealth.com. https://www.everydayhealth.com/diet-and-nutrition/diet/tips-weight-loss-actually-work/

Office of Dietary Supplements - Dietary Supplements for Immune Function and Infectious Diseases. (n.d.). https://ods.od.nih.gov/factsheets/ImmuneFunction-HealthProfessional/

Morey, J. N., Boggero, I. A., Scott, A. B., & Segerstrom, S. C. (2015, October). Current directions in stress and human immune function. *Current Opinion in Psychology*, *5*, 13–17. https://doi.org/10.1016/j.copsyc.2015.03.007

Made in United States
Troutdale, OR
02/14/2024

17674679R00116